Beauty Pure and Simple

Beauty Pure and Simple

The Ayurvedic Approach to Beautiful Skin

Kristen Ma

TRUMPETER
Boston & London 2011

Trumpeter Books
An imprint of Shambhala Publications, Inc.
Horticultural Hall
300 Massachusetts Avenue
Boston, Massachusetts 02115
trumpeterbooks.com

9 8 7 6 5 4 3 2 1

First Edition
Printed in the United States of America
⊗This edition is printed on acid-free paper that meets the American
National Standards Institute z39.48 Standard.
♻This book is printed on 30% postconsumer recycled paper. For
more information please visit us at www.shambhala.com.
Distributed in the United States by Random House, Inc.,
and in Canada by Random House of Canada Ltd

Library of Congress Cataloging-in-Publication Data

Ma, Kristen.
Beauty pure and simple: the ayurvedic approach to beautiful skin /
Kristen Ma.—1st ed.
p.   cm.
Includes index.
ISBN 978-1-59030-920-9 (pbk.: acid-free paper)
1. Skin—Care and hygiene. 2. Medicine, Ayurvedic. I. Title.
RL87.M214 2011
646.7'2—dc23
2011014502

Contents

Acknowledgments

As with all the successes in my life, I have to thank many people for their contributions and support:

My mother, Jean, who has provided me with so much opportunity. Your vata energy has kept the momentum and movement of this project going.

Dr. Vasant Lad, Dr. Subhash Ranade, Dr. Avinash Lele, and Dr. Jeson Yan, who taught and inspired me to transform my view of health, skin, and love.

Dr. T. G. Lewis, who has encouraged me so much and always emphasized the importance of discipline. I especially thank you for educating me about the importance of breathing.

Lindsey Simms, Yvonne Kurant, Peter Howie, and Alison Sherk, who are not only coworkers but good friends who generously gave me their time and feedback.

My partner, Benjamin, who has cooled my most heated, frustrated moments with his kindness and patience.

The Pure + simple staff, all of them talented and educated practitioners and coordinators, who have helped me learn so much about beauty and team building.

Introduction

In this competitive modern age, we have high expectations. Not only do we demand top performance from products, services, and technologies, but we also demand it of ourselves. Most of us strive to be the best in our jobs, in our relationships, and as members of our communities. Naturally, our attitude toward how we look is just as uncompromising. We demand ourselves to have flawless skin and hard bodies, believing physical perfection is always within our complete control. This gives way to frustration with ourselves when we don't achieve this often unrealistic goal.

But by placing such expectations on ourselves, we sometimes forget what beauty really is and how best to embody it. As an esthetician, I see two different sides to the promotion of beauty. One emphasizes traits like glowing skin, shiny hair, bright eyes, and a strong body, which can only come from balanced health that makes us innately magnetic and disarming.

Unfortunately, the other side of beauty promotion has nothing to do with health; it focuses on a straight or small nose, big breasts, pouty lips, and taut skin. It rigidly supports the idea that beauty can be attained synthetically through fake nails, fake hair, a fake tan, and fake eyelashes. This emphasis on external perfection over well-being leads to the use of dangerous procedures that damage rather than enhance health, especially that of the skin.

It was this dichotomy that led my mother, Jean Eng, and I to start Pure + simple, Inc., which comprises a chain of holistic spas and a line of natural skin care products and mineral makeup. Our mandate was to offer alternatives to conventional products and treatments to promote beauty through health. These alternatives included both chemical-free skin care and skin consultations with estheticians that emphasized inside-outside beauty. After a few years of operation, I decided to strengthen my understanding of the connection between health and beauty by becoming an ayurvedic practitioner.

Ayurveda, the five-thousand-year-old Indian science of health and medicine, teaches that healing (and therefore beauty) stems from a balanced lifestyle supported by knowledge. It is based on the concept that our bodies are composed of three different energies: *pitta*, heat energy; *kapha*, water and earth energy; and *vata*, air and space energy. It is not the breakdown of our physical systems that causes sickness, but an excess or a deficiency of a specific energy that unbalances and compromises our total selves.

One principle that runs consistently through all Eastern medicine is the idea that we must participate in our own well-being instead of hoping for someone or something else to save us. Whether it is a drug, a surgical procedure, or a practitioner, many of us expect an external intervention to heal us, giving little thought to how we ourselves contribute to our health status and recovery. This principle also applies to beauty. Ayurveda promotes a more proactive approach, emphasizing prevention instead of short-term solutions that merely suppress symptoms. Many people suffer from acne, rosacea, eczema, hyperpigmentation, and premature aging, which may seem like ugly nuisances but can, in fact, be early warning signs of more serious problems. Using these imperfections as a spur to change can result not only in beautiful skin but in better health and greater vitality.

In particular, ayurveda relies on daily care to deal with unsightly symptoms by addressing their underlying cause. In contrast, current Western culture often encourages neglect of this responsibility, opting instead for acute, drastic treatments in pursuit of false ideals. These harsh procedures—intended to reduce fine lines, tone, and even reconstruct features—are often counterproductive, because they tax our bodies, minds, emotions, and immune systems. We must see beauty as something we want to develop naturally from the inside out.

The repercussions of treating skin severely can be long-lasting. The skin is a delicate organ with its own internal system. Although many people think it consists of only what they see, it is actually composed of three layers of tissue, each with its own sublayers. Together they encapsulate a network of capillaries and sweat glands bound by tightly woven fibers of collagen and elastin. Understanding how complex and fragile our skin is can help us make more informed choices.

My clientele is made up of people who did not initially have this understanding and who made rash decisions with the help of medical professionals. Many have adult skin conditions that are a direct result of having treated teenage acne with harsh peels, medications, and drying agents prescribed by dermatologists or other physicians. These solutions typically produced short-term, temporary results and long-term damage such as skin sensitivity, dehydration, and mental stress.

I, too, treated my skin badly. I suffered from acne for more than ten years and desperately searched for a solution, spending endless amounts of money and energy on my stubbornly blemished face. I tried dry ice, glycolic peels, and salicylic acid, all of which made my skin red and created scars that I still have today. When none of these methods worked, I took antibiotics, which not only made me feel ill but also caused dehydration.

I often compare this struggle to a war. I was fighting the acne as if it were an external enemy and not a part of me. It was only when I started to treat it with natural skin care methods that I began to see a difference. Though I hadn't really believed such a simple solution would be effective, I had exhausted most other avenues and was willing to try anything.

At first, I achieved only a lessening of my skin's redness, but in time, my whole face began to look healthier. While I still had blemishes, they looked less irritated. This motivated me to shift from using "oil-free" and "purifying" products to natural, nourishing ones that targeted sensitivity and dehydration. My skin finally became more balanced, and I began to break out less. At that point, I was inspired to take responsibility for my overall health by conducting a series of detoxes and dietary changes.

This journey led me to love natural beauty care. Not only did I clear up my skin and increase my self-confidence, but I learned how to treat myself gently and love myself. Now, along with more attractive skin, I have a new perspective on myself and on how both the mind and the inner workings of the body affect the skin. I only wish I had learned these things earlier!

The reason many of us make mistakes when choosing our health and beauty care is that we are driven by fear: fear that we are not attractive, that people don't like us, that we cannot achieve our goals. According to ayurveda, fear not only affects the function of our kidneys, but it also prevents us from moving forward with a positive attitude. Today, critical events in our world and the environment require us to act. We need to feel empowered, and that feeling can only come from knowledge, because knowledge *is* power.

When I was growing up, my mother always said, "Kristen, people can steal your things—your car, your watch, even your husband—but they can't take away what's in your mind. Knowledge and wisdom are your most important investments." But acquiring knowledge about how to treat the skin can be difficult. There is so much information on cosmetics and skin care products to wade through, and a lot of it is conflicting. Despite all the clutter from the promotion of various lotions and potions online and at department stores, spas, and drugstores, we often are not told what we really need to know, such as which products contain caustic or even toxic ingredients.

When my mother and I first launched Pure + simple a decade ago, natural skin care was not in vogue. We had to do a lot of educating, and many of our clients were initially skeptical. However, as more of them saw tangible results in their complexions and passed the word to others, the demand for our services and products flourished.

Avoiding harmful ingredients and choosing healthy ones is only part of the solution. At Pure + simple, we believe in coupling natural skin care with a balanced lifestyle. Through this book, I want to help others care for themselves in a way that allows them to feel beautiful and vibrant—and have glowing skin. I hope that, armed with a healthy approach to self-image, people will be able to reexamine their outlook and emphasize the positive, so we can all make effective changes in our lives and in the world. Many clients have already told me that Pure + simple has changed their lives. I'm honored and encouraged to hear this, because I intend to go beyond merely promoting wonderful skin care to teaching the proven knowledge and intuition of ayurveda. By listening to our bodies and choosing appropriate actions, we can look and feel our best. Nothing is more attractive than a self-empowered person who is healthy in mind, body, and spirit.

We at Pure + simple are modernists with a practical, realistic outlook. While we promote natural skin care, we know that people have different goals and face unique challenges. When our clients resort to chemical medications or invasive surgeries, we use our knowledge to help them compensate for side effects and unforeseen consequences in the best way possible, because we believe that being judgmental or uncompromising is also unhealthy.

Everything on earth can be a poison or a cure, depending on what and who we are treating. For example, in contrast to popular Western belief, Eastern medicine teaches that some of us benefit from the stimulation of smoking and the heaviness of starchy carbohydrates, while others cannot take the overstimulation of regular cardio exercise. Balance is everything. This philosophy extends to how we view beauty treatments. While many purists insist that basic facials and good creams are enough to heal any skin ailment, we believe that some aggressive, yet noninvasive procedures, if done conscientiously, can be extremely beneficial. This is especially true for those looking for anti-aging results.

Modern procedures like intense pulsed light (IPL) therapy, light-emitting diode (LED) treatments, and sea-salt microdermabrasion can eliminate spots of hyperpigmentation and the visible effects of broken capillaries, as well as minimize fine lines. Skin care and massage alone cannot yield the results of these more stimulating treatments. Proper selection and customization make these methods truly effective. Pairing new technology with the ancient methodology of choosing skin care treatments and products based on each person's ayurvedic constitution is the basis of Pure + simple's approach.

A friend of mine, who is a computer programmer, once told me, "Compared to the human body, computers are easy. They simply code zeros and ones in different patterns, whereas our bodies have so many complex systems!" I was surprised at this viewpoint, because I'm so often frustrated by my computer. My friend made me realize how often we see technology as sophisticated while taking our own amazing capacities for granted. When I was studying at the Ayurvedic Institute in New Mexico, its founder and principle instructor, Dr. Vasant Lad, told our class that the more he learned about the way our bodies worked, the more he believed in God: who else could create such a perfect and intricate system?

Our bodies are worlds within worlds. Each is a holistic system containing seven interconnected subordinate systems: circulatory, nervous, endocrine, muscular, lymphatic, digestive, and skeletal. It is this complexity that makes knowing what is healthy so difficult. And since each person is a unique individual, no one solution can be good for everyone. That is why I always tell my clients they are the experts when it comes to themselves. They have been with themselves twenty-four hours a day for their whole lives. My job is simply to listen and provide additional knowledge and support.

I found my own search for health and beauty exasperating because different experts touted different studies and opinions about what was good and bad. I got to the point where I couldn't eat anything or follow any regimen without second-guessing myself. Simply sustaining myself became overwhelming. By writing this book, I hope to make my own hard-won knowledge available as a tool and a resource for others who are interested in holistic, natural ways. Along with normal skin care and maintenance, we will discuss the three basic principles that can apply to everything from the search for beauty to emotional exploration: moving, purging, and nourishing. For reformed skin abusers, I will also explain how to repair existing damage and the best ways to treat ailments like acne, sensitivity, rosacea, eczema, hyperpigmentation, and signs of aging (tissue degeneration). This book is a compilation of knowledge that we at Pure + simple wish to pass on to those of you who, at present, are just browsing, in hopes that you too will be inspired to embrace the ayurvedic process of beautification.

Many of my clients came to Pure + simple as beauty refugees searching for a positive and healthy way to look and feel good. We offer a more nurturing option than traditional methods: skin care that is gentle and nourishing, made from pure ingredients, along with knowledge that fosters positive choices.

Part One

A TIMELESS PHILOSOPHY OF BEAUTY

One

Natural Skin Care Explained

There has been a lot of hype about natural and organic beauty products, but what exactly are the benefits? Why go natural? Why spend the extra money and effort to sort through the cluttered world of cosmetics? How can you tell which product lines are actually natural and which are just capitalizing on the trend?

During my years in the beauty industry, I have seen the changes my clients have achieved with natural skin care compared to those who use chemical brands, and it is astounding. Some people assume that natural ingredients will be less potent, but my own battle with acne showed me firsthand that chemical-based skin care brands do not produce sustainable, long-term beauty solutions.

Natural Skin Care for a More Beautiful Complexion

The goal of using skin care is simple: to enhance and support the attractiveness of your skin. If you don't get visible results, there is no point in using a product. While we will discuss the importance of avoiding toxic chemicals for overall health, it is essential to emphasize the benefits that natural products have for your complexion. When you use products without pore-clogging synthetic bases or drying chemical detergents, you let your skin maintain balance and reap the therapeutic benefits of wholesome, natural ingredients.

Let's start with discussing the beautifying properties of skin care that contains a completely natural base. Because the base makes up the bulk of a product, it's the most important aspect to assess. Natural products use pure vegetable and plant oils, waters, and waxes as their base, whereas conventional product lines use petroleum (mineral oil, petrolatum, propylene glycol, and so on). Skin loves (and easily absorbs) natural ingredients; conversely, it does not like petrochemicals. It acts as a gatekeeper to limit their harmful effects, which is why using natural skin care helps prevent pore congestion. Since petroleum molecules are too large to fully absorb, products that contain petrochemicals clog pores and suffocate the skin. This causes outbreaks of acne and blackheads, preventing the skin from accepting moisture from both skin care products and the humidity in the air.

This realization often provides a eureka moment for my clients who have tried countless moisturizers only to have them sit on the skin's surface without proper penetration. One client, a PhD biochemistry student, came to Pure + simple frustrated after exploring everything from the science of hormones to high-tech peels. She had spent a great deal of money and tried many approaches, none of which had cured her acne. Her dermatologist had given her medicated creams containing benzoyl peroxide and salicylic acid, which dried out her skin, making it flaky and irritated in addition to the blemishes. Her dry, sensitive skin was being further dehydrated by these acne-targeting products that unbalanced her oil production and clogged her pores.

During her first consultation, I explained how natural ingredients are absorbed, then prescribed a gentle, restorative regime consisting of multiple moisturizers and an anti-inflammatory face oil. Being the goal-oriented young woman she was, she purchased all of the recommended products, though I was unsure if she was truly convinced. To my surprise, she returned with flowers to thank me for changing her understanding of beauty care. Her skin had responded right away, and today she is completely acne-free. She attributes this improvement to daily use of an oil-rich, moisturizing cream mask that has helped repair her skin and therefore reduce irritation and sensitivity. The success she experienced was the combination of reduced pore congestion and nourishment from her natural skin care routine.

A truly natural product should be one that is packed full of replenishing, pure ingredients. Unfortunately, some companies combine a few natural ingredients with a lot of water and chemical-based thickeners instead of using completely natural formulations. This means the product has very few healing properties. A totally natural regimen must contain nutritious ingredients that fully penetrate the skin to nourish and restore it and protect it against further damage. It is crucial to understand that the skin is a delicate organ that needs to be pampered and handled with care in order to regenerate properly. Although many people consider this fact when treating sensitive or dehydrated skin, they may not know that it also applies to acne-prone skin.

Being gentle, through the use of natural ingredients and cleansers, is one of the best ways to maintain a clear complexion. Contrary to popular belief, stripping the skin is actually a contributor to breakouts and blackheads. This is why natural cleansers are so important. Harsh chemical detergents in conventional skin care products deplete the skin's acid mantle—the coating of sebum on its surface, which is made up of fatty acids, alcohol, waxes, salts, and lactic acid. This mantle creates a barrier against bacteria, so overcleansing and stripping decreases its resilience, leaving it damaged and prone to reactions like infection and oil imbalance. The more we deplete our skin of its natural oils, the more sebum (oil) it produces in an attempt to maintain proper protection. This additional oil, coupled with the dehydration caused by chemical detergents, fosters the perfect environment for clogged pores. Instead of sebum flowing over the skin as a dewy, lubricating barrier, it becomes trapped in dried-out oil deposits that inhibit the absorption of moisture and promote blemishes.

Whether your problem is pores clogged from petroleum buildup or an imbalance caused by harsh cleansers and nutrient-poor skin care products, avoiding chemicals and choosing skin care made with rejuvenating, natural ingredients is the fastest way to flawless, beautiful skin.

Natural Skin Care for Wellness Inside and Out

I was never very interested in working in the beauty industry until I understood its link to wellness. Although I found grooming the perfect brow and shaping graceful nails to be fun, these esthetics on their own were not something to which I wanted to devote my life. The broader picture—teaching people how to love themselves and be more conscious of their bodies—was what I really wanted to endorse.

In my opinion, beauty is much more than skin deep. True beauty is the reflection of a healthy mind and body, because there is nothing more attractive than someone who radiates vitality. Unfortunately, the use of conventional chemical skin care can actually tax the body.

While this may sound radical, it is important to understand that all products applied to the skin are absorbed into the bloodstream and internal organs. Therefore, products containing toxic chemicals will affect overall health. Sunscreens, makeup, and skin care products are often made with dangerous ingredients that eventually damage your health in ways you would never suspect. For example, certain cosmetic preservatives are identified carcinogens; sunscreen agents mimic estrogen and unbalance the hormonal system; and chemicals used as bases for almost all products tax the kidneys and liver. Yet we apply products containing these additives to our skin on a regular basis.

It is not only the contents of the products we use with which we need to be concerned; we must also be aware of their packaging. Various plastics can leave residue or leach toxicity into products, making the use of glass and food-grade plastics extremely important. Remember, all of the principles we apply to skin care ingredients also apply to any materials that interact with them. This is why many companies need to become much more holistic in their product development and design. Ceramic and glass packaging is not only more resilient, but it also maintains the purity of the product. Because these materials do not degrade as easily and are less porous than weaker materials (like plastic), they may allow the use of less potent, more natural preservatives as well. Moreover, glass and ceramics are reusable and more sustainable, which is also better for the environment.

Natural Skin Care to Encourage Social Responsibility

Personal beauty is only fulfilling when we also encourage beauty in our environment. Being beautiful inside and out means being conscious of how we consume and what ideas we promote. Our ideas on beauty greatly reflect who we are and what beliefs we hold. How we behave as individuals has a larger impact than simply giving lip service to our principles. Working for ethical companies and buying socially responsible products makes a powerful statement about how we view the environment, and this crosses over into our skin care decisions.

Biodegradable products have a synergy with the earth. What we wash from our body or eliminate, we put into the world's ecosystem. Antidepressants, hormones, and plasticides, passed through people as waste, have been found in public water supplies. This was noted in the

1980s when fish species in the Saint Lawrence River began to display gender changes. Certain fish were found to have both eggs and testes. A study in which they were fed to lab rats showed that, over time, the rats also displayed hormone imbalances. We must realize what an impact our consumption has on the ecosystem.

But respecting the planet does not have to mean letting go of our desire for beautiful skin; instead, it requires us to support companies that produce skin care products responsibly. Many vertically integrated natural skin care companies actually farm their ingredients respectfully by giving their land a cyclical rest so as not to deplete its fertility. Others go a step further and make use of biodynamic farming, which entails replenishing the soil and refraining from the use of pesticides that would disturb natural insect life. The traditional agricultural practices involved actually build carbon back into the soil.

As mentioned earlier, we need to consider packaging when making shopping decisions. The environmentalist Paul Hawken said, "Any time someone steals something from our future, it is injustice. . . . We steal from the future and sell it in the present and call it GDP [gross domestic product]." Packaging is not only wasteful; it can also affect the safety of a product. At Pure + simple, we limit the amount of packaging for each product and use renewable materials. For example, the compacts in our cosmetic line are refillable so the compact itself can be reused and the makeup replaced as needed. We also use glass containers for our skin care products, because glass maintains purity and is a more sustainable material. For items that cannot be stored in glass (such as those used in the shower), we use squeeze bottles made of 100 percent postconsumer materials. We also have a bottle-return service (as more and more companies do), through which we wash, sterilize, and reuse bottles, cutting costs as well as waste.

As consumers, we must realize that industrial pollution is no longer acceptable business practice, and we can communicate this by making more conscious buying decisions. Promoting positive ideas and business practices is the first step in changing counterproductive social habits. Buying natural skin care endorses businesses that put the health of their customers first.

I want to emphasize that I am not referring only to physical health. It is important that we promote a healthy, practical perception of beauty in our society, because the current definitions of beauty can be very dysfunctional. Many women and men engage in unhealthy and irresponsible behavior due to poor self-image and the pressure to conform to modern interpretations of beauty. We must stop wishing we were someone else; pining for the perfect cheekbones, lips, hips, and breasts; and believing that artificial enhancements are the answer. Loving and accepting our humanness instead of fixating on our supposed imperfections is integral to developing a healthy outlook. Cosmetic companies that help their clients enhance their natural beauty foster such acceptance and make the concept of beauty attainable for everyone. These values are worthy of support and patronage.

A truly natural and holistic beauty company helps to increase self-awareness in its community, urging people to become more in tune with the changes in their bodies. I continually encourage my clients to notice what happens to their breathing and heart rate when they experience stress; I teach them to change their skin care when the weather changes; and I also offer dietary advice. When people learn to use diet, skin care, and stress relief to balance their bodies, they become more aware of how to monitor their health. They also become more aware of and empowered by the relationship between mind, body, emotions, and environment.

What Is Natural Skin Care?

Now that you know how important using natural skin care can be, you're ready to skip out and buy new pure products, right? All you have to do is throw out all of your chemical-based cosmetics and re-stock your medicine cabinet with those that proudly tout the words *natural* or *organic*. If only it were that easy!

Unfortunately, many of us find that the search for truly natural skin care can be difficult, because defining what *natural* means can be confusing. The definition of natural skin care products has become clouded. A company can label its products natural if they contain as little as 2 percent natural ingredients, as this is the minimum required by US law. Unfortunately, consumers assume that this labeling ensures completely natural content.

For obvious reasons, real standards of natural products are needed, but because the beauty industry is unregulated, the definitions must come from us. Luckily, many natural skin care companies are beginning to put their own standards in place, most including three main parameters.

First, a truly natural product must contain at least 95 percent fully natural ingredients that remain in their natural state and have not been highly processed. To determine whether a product has a high chemical content, check the package for International Nomenclature of Cosmetic Ingredients (INCI) labeling. Such labeling gives the scientific names for ingredients and help identify a cosmetic's true content. Some products use vague terms such as "vegetable-based cleansing agent," but INCI names let you properly identify the specific origins of an ingredient and often how it is produced. INCI names are easily deciphered by online cosmetic ingredient databases such as the Skin Deep database (cosmetic sdatabase.com) run by The Environmental Working Group.

The second parameter is that manufacturing should not significantly or adversely alter the purity or effect of the natural ingredients. The natural ingredients need to be extracted and preserved naturally as well. Some certification organizations, such as Ecocert, assess manufacturers' production methods for any risk of contamination as well as those for a product's packaging. This helps consumers easily understand a product's standards. Ecocert requires items to not be packaged in PVC or polystyrene as they can leach into products. All certified items must be packaged in nonpolluting, recyclable containers. But keep in mind that seals and certifications can be extremely expensive and thus cost-prohibitive for smaller companies that may be high-quality producers. By checking INCI labels and researching a company's values and inquiring about the origins of its products' ingredients, we can make more informed decisions. Transparency is a good indication of authenticity.

Finally, natural products must contain no ingredients that have a potential or suspected health risk. Since the point of natural skin care products is the betterment of both our skin and well-being, health safety is important. While this may sound like simple logic, many ingredients commonly found in skin, body, and hair care products are carcinogenic, toxic, or identified endocrine (hormone) disrupters.

INGREDIENTS TO AVOID

While there are many harmful chemical ingredients in our beauty products, the two I find myself discussing most often are petrolatum and sodium laurel sulfate (SLS), simply because they are the most ubiquitous.

Petrolatum (also known as petroleum jelly and many other names), a petroleum by-product, is used as a cosmetic base and can be found in almost all skin care, cosmetics, and hair products. All petrochemicals are extremely detrimental to our health, and because petrolatum is used as a base, it makes up a huge portion of any given product. Unlike harmful synthetic preservatives and additives, which usually account for a very low percentage of the formulation (but must also be avoided), petrolatum and other petrochemicals are present in large quantities.

When checking to see what is in those mysterious bottles of skin care goop, you will find it is mainly petrolatum, a few additives, and a lot of water. The main cosmetic-related problem with petrolatum or paraffinium (petroleum) is that its molecules are too large to fully penetrate the skin. Therefore, products made with it sit on the skin surface, clogging the pores. Early in my career, while working at an elite spa in Sydney, Australia, I ran out of the petroleum jelly we used to protect the delicate skin around the eyes while doing a lash tint. I was told to substitute a very expensive brand of neck cream. I realized that this high-end neck cream was simply dressed-up petroleum jelly! It would not absorb into the skin; it would just sit on the surface and act as a barrier.

Petroleum is also used as a barrier in antiperspirants. Containing both aluminum and petroleum, antiperspirant sticks keep the moisture from the suderiferous (sweat) glands from reaching the skin surface.

Petroleum dehydrates the skin, which is ironic, since it is used as the base for most moisturizers. Though many of these moisturizers feature wonderful ingredients (antioxidants, vitamins, and so on), they cannot be fully absorbed into the skin. Using petroleum on your skin is like masking your face with plastic wrap. While it makes an excellent barrier for acute situations (against windburn while skiing, for example), it is unhealthy when used on a daily basis. Many people, myself included, have self-induced acne by applying petroleum-based products; the pore congestion contributes to blackheads and blemishes. These products can also irritate sensitive skin and trigger allergies.

Petroleum also presents internal dangers. What little does absorb into the skin has been found to cause kidney damage and liver abnormalities. It is the same basic material as gasoline, and people apply it to their faces, bodies, and scalps. Besides the direct harm to the human body, petrochemicals take vast amounts of energy to produce and are nonrenewable, so they also hurt the environment.

Sodium laurel sulfate is a harsh detergent mostly found in products such as facial cleanser, shampoo, soap, toothpaste, astringent, and toner. It has a foaming property and gives the skin that tight feeling many equate with being "deeply cleansed." In fact, SLS disturbs the skin's acid mantle and strips it of its natural oils. This is especially detrimental for sensitive skin and leads to rosacea, eczema, and dermatitis.

The body is always working to attain balance and heal. When we use products with SLS, the body attempts to balance out the dryness the chemical creates by producing more oil; therefore, SLS dehydrates aging skin and stimulates oil production in the sebaceous glands of oily skin. The now-overactive glands pour out sebum (oil) to compensate for the skin's dehydration.

Sodium laurel sulfate may also cause internal damage. It is absorbed by delicate mouth tissues from toothpaste and through the scalp via shampoos and conditioners. Once absorbed, it is retained in the internal organs. Because it strips skin of its natural defenses, it increases the absorption of other toxic materials, making the body more vulnerable to disease. Studies have also shown that SLS combines with various cosmetic ingredients to create carcinogenic nitrates and dioxin. It is thought to retard healing and promote tissue malformation.

Petrolatum and SLS are not the only harmful chemicals to avoid. Others include the following:

Propylene and butylene glycol: These petroleum-derived ingredients are used in skin and hair products to temporarily boost skin hydration. Long term, they can dehydrate and damage skin and hair structure.

Like similar chemicals, they can cause kidney damage and liver abnormalities.

Carbomer: A petroleum-derived thickener, carbomer helps mask the fact that a product may be composed mostly of water instead of skin-nourishing ingredients. It is commonly used in creams, bath products, and eye makeup.

Sunscreen agents: Some chemical sunscreen agents—such as benzophenone-3 and octyl methoxycinnamate—mimic estrogen, confusing the endocrine system. In contrast, mineral sunblocks, like zinc oxide and titanium, are natural materials that reduce photoactivity.

Parabens (including butylparaben, methylparaben, and propylparaben): Parabens are a formaldehyde-derived group of preservatives used in cosmetics and food. They mimic estrogen and have been cited as carcinogens.

Cortisone: Cortisone is a steroid used for its anti-inflammatory effects. Over time, it thins the skin and weakens its immune response. It also suppresses the body's normal immune response. Dermatologists often prescribe cortisone creams to soothe eczema, acne, and general inflammation.

Phthalates: A group of liquid chemicals resembling oil, phthalates are used as fixatives to slow evaporation—making the scent in perfumes and other products linger—and as plasticizers in nail polish. Phthalates are endocrine disrupters and carcinogens. They have been shown to cause blood clots, along with damage to the heart and lungs.

Coal tar: Used to manufacture commercial dyes and industrial paints, coal tar is also an ingredient in color cosmetics, hair dyes, and makeup. It is a known carcinogen and may make skin more sensitive to sunlight.

Diethanolamine (DEA): Diethanolamine is used as a wetting and foaming agent in shampoos and body washes and to preserve the texture of lotions and creams. It becomes unsafe when it reacts with nitrites in other products, forming nitrosamines and possibly becoming a carcinogen. DEA is also an endocrine disruptor.

Diazolidinyl urea and imidazolidinyl urea: These common preservatives in cosmetics release formaldehyde. They are known carcinogens, and they can trigger allergies. They can also cause contact dermatitis and headaches.

Knowing what ingredients are used in grooming products and cosmetics is extremely important if you want to care properly for your skin, body, and overall health. Natural skin care respects the delicacy of your skin and means that only wholesome, pure ingredients will be absorbed into your body.

We cannot discount the interconnectedness of our well-being. Our skin is so much more than what we see on the surface. It is part of our overall body system, and its beauty is reflected in a balance which is found much deeper within us. Real, effective skin care is the pairing of a healthy, toxin-free regimen with close attention to the well-being of body, mind, and spirit.

Two

Ayurveda: The Beauty of Eastern Medicine

I only truly began to understand what natural beauty meant when I discovered ayurveda. I believe this ancient science is helpful in our pursuit of flawless skin, because it is a health system that is both preventive and holistic. Most healing methods, whether conventional or alternative, fail to offer a usable, consistent system that empowers the patient. Ayurveda's framework is so simple that everyone can make daily choices for balancing their health in relation to their specific environment, health, and personal needs. The spiritual dimension of ayurveda also offers a philosophy of beauty that profoundly supports and develops the mind, body, and spirit.

Ayurveda literally translates to "the science/study of life." Dating back five thousand years to the Himalayans in northern India, it guides followers to live in harmony and beauty, according to their individual constitutions and environment. It bases its treatments on how people have unique needs, perspectives, personalities, metabolic rates, and so on. Therefore, it is logical that each of us must customize our treatment, diet, and habits in order to maintain health, feel beautiful, and live with vitality.

Since ayurveda emphasizes prevention, we learn to become self-aware through listening to ourselves—our intuition and our body. Treating small imbalances can prevent an accumulation of problems that can lead to disease, but this requires us to be responsible and pro-active in our wellness care and to take an active role in our healing.

In India, ayurvedic doctors are traditionally paid an annual fixed fee for each patient rather than on a case-by-case basis (sometimes they are simply paid whatever a patient can offer). Since treating sicker patients requires more time and energy, this system encourages a pro-active, preventive approach. Not only are these physicians healers, but they are also teachers who educate their patients on maintaining health and preventing disease. While Western surgeons are highly compensated for treating severe situations, ayurvedic doctors are rewarded for avoiding invasive procedures.

Ayurveda also has an entire branch of posttreatment rejuvenation that uses therapies and medicines to restore the body and its tissues after the trauma of surgery. This highlights not only the importance of recovery in ayurveda but also the role of beauty, since the *rasayanas* (herbs and practices used for rejuvenation) are prescribed to support the skin and body as they age. Herbs such as ashwagandha; and practices such as full-body oiling are common examples of rasayanas. Because the herbs and practices like these bolster the immune system and increase tissue regeneration, this facet of ayurveda is also a wonderful, holistic form of antiaging.

Ayurveda is an incredibly romantic ideology. It encompasses love, sex, and beauty as part of a healthy lifestyle. Caring for the skin and body is a daily ayurvedic ritual, beginning with a morning self-massage followed by cleansing and exfoliation with ayurvedic herbs. Beauty rituals are not seen as a form of recreation; they are ways to learn more about yourself, tend and care for your body, and give you an opportunity to notice the subtle changes that occur within you.

According to ayurveda, the key to understanding your health (and hence your means to gorgeous skin) is in perceiving that everything about your mind, body, and environment is always changing. This means that your rituals and products must also change to accommodate this state of perpetual flux; what is good for one season is not good for another, and the skin care and diet you followed five years ago may no longer suit your current needs. Finding harmony and grounding within constant change is the key to both happiness and beauty.

I can provide only a snapshot of ayurveda in this book, as it is a vast ideology with many facets; however, I will explain its basic principles to help you develop a deeper understanding of health, balance, and beauty.

How Is Ayurveda Different from Western Medicine?

Western (allopathic) medicine often focuses on alleviating symptoms and treating pain, inflammation, tumors, or depression with narcotics, anti-inflammatories, antidepressants, and surgery. This approach ignores the source of the dysfunction or disease, which is parallel to our approach to beauty. Western treatments try to minimize wrinkles, dry out pimples, and cover or camouflage redness without seeking out the lifestyle and behavior imbalances that create these symptoms.

Ayurveda, in contrast, searches for the root cause of a given ailment and treats imbalance and disease from this perspective. It examines diet, sleeping patterns, thoughts, emotions, and behavior. Going even further, it assesses the state of a person's energies (or *doshas*).

According to ayurveda, to understand ourselves as individuals, we must first determine our constitution by looking at *doshas*. Doshas are the energetic elements we all possess: kapha is the earth/water dosha; pitta is the fire dosha; and vata is the air dosha. The doshas are the basic building blocks of who we are, and we each have a unique combination of them. While Western medicine looks at how individual organs and systems are working, ayurveda considers the quality of our doshas much more important. Although this concept seems abstract, it is actually quite simple.

Each dosha is represented by its element (or elements). To find the real source of a particular condition, we examine what is happening with our subtle elemental energy—whether or not our doshas are functioning properly or are in balance. Sometimes we feel we are suffering from many different ailments, when in fact they are all governed by the same dosha. Once this dosha is put back in balance with the proper herbs, diet, and lifestyle choices, many of our health concerns clear up. Our symptoms indicate what is happening within us; a solution or cure comes from addressing our kapha, pitta, and/or vata.

The kapha dosha is embodied by earth and water. It is responsible for everything within the body that is moist, solid, stable, and capable of growth and retention. Mucus is produced by kapha energy, lubricating and moisturizing passages and internal organs. Because the lungs are kapha organs, an excess of kapha in the system means an overproduction of mucus and resulting respiratory problems. Every increase in and accumulation of tissue is also related to kapha. Too much kapha energy results in weight gain, water retention, cyst formation, and skin tags (growths).

Pitta is the fire dosha and demonstrates this element through heat and inflammation. It governs digestion because, like fire, it cooks and assimilates our food into nutrients. Too much pitta energy leads to symptoms such as hyperacidity, heartburn, ulcers, or acid reflux. Since pitta is related to all inflammation, it is also responsible for blood cell matter (specifically red blood cells). Overactive pitta translates into skin sensitivity and redness caused by dilated capillaries and overstimulated circulation.

Vata, the air dosha, governs all spaces and hollows within the body. Like wind, it also dictates the action of movement. This is why vata is in charge of the nervous system, sending intangible messages throughout the body. Spurred by the quality of air, vata possesses the characteristic of dryness. Excess vata creates dryness, but even when it is in balance, vata is dry in quality. The kidneys, which regulate water metabolism, are vata organs, and when they become overworked and exhausted, creating excess vata energy, they cause dehydration in the body and skin.

The concept of doshas is important, because it emphasizes an important difference between Western medicine and ayurveda: each individual is unique and must be healed uniquely. Western physicians use the same drugs and methods to treat everyone who has the same symptoms, but in ayurveda, healing depends on the person and his or her natural doshic constitution.

We are born with all three doshas within us, but it is the degree of each dosha that makes us unique. Usually one will be dominant with the other two exerting a lesser influence. However, some people have two main doshas, and rare individuals are tridoshic, meaning they have equal amounts of all three. Once you know who you are from a doshic standpoint, you can understand the imbalances to which you are prone. You begin to see and feel when your body is out of balance, diverting you from your natural, optimal state.

The Three Doshas: Kapha, Pitta, Vata

Now that we have talked about the concept of ayurveda and the doshas, let's look at each dosha in more depth. This will allow you to identify which of these energies are dominant in your body.

KAPHA: EARTH AND WATER

Those with strong kapha have an abundance of water and earth energy. And like water and earth, Kapha governs moisture, solidness, heaviness, and coldness. Kapha represents growth, nutrients, and their storage. Physically, kaphas are slow-moving and fleshy with large, heavy-boned frames. Women are often voluptuous, while men are inclined to be husky and develop muscle easily. Their features are full and substantial, their nails strong and hard. Kapha skin is thick and oily with a predisposition to enlarged pores, but if hydrated and healthy, the complexion can appear flawless. Kaphas are often considered classically beautiful, as they possess large, radiant eyes; broad and prominent noses; full lips; and luxuriant hair. They also tend to be the healthiest, most robust of the dosha types, as they have everything in abundance, including stamina and strong immune systems.

Kaphas' health problems arise from that quality of abundance, since they have a tendency to gain weight—a genetic trait reinforced by their habits. They may also suffer from sinus congestion (accumulation of mucus), edema (accumulation and retention of water), candida (accumulation of fungus), and cystic acne (accumulation of toxins and oil).

Kaphas' physical qualities of heaviness, moistness, abundance, and retention are also reflected in their personalities. They are routine-oriented, grounded, nurturing, loyal, and dependable. They have excellent knowledge retention and are sentimental about holding on to tradition. They can also be incredibly romantic and sensuous lovers, since they understand the importance of taking the time to enjoy each moment.

Character flaws for kaphas who are out of balance follow this same theme of abundance. They are inclined toward greed, neediness, and self-indulgence (accumulation of wealth, inability to let go, overeating, and so on) and can be resistant to change (lack of flexibility). Those with an unhealthy excess of kapha are also lethargic and depressive.

While the kapha body type and temperament are not often cele-brated in our modern media, it is something to be cherished and appre-ciated. For it is the kapha ability to be still and stable, that is necessary to achieve the peace and serenity of nirvana.

Pitta: Fire

Pitta individuals are characterized by the fire dosha. This dosha's quali-ties are hot, sharp, and light. Pitta governs transformation, just as fire creates heat and heat causes chemical changes. It is the pitta dosha that is responsible for transformations in the body such as metabolism (transforming stored fat to energy), digestion (transforming food to energy), and cellular transformation.

Physically, pitta is manifested in a medium, athletic build of average height. Pittas embody heat with sensitive skin that can also be prone to allergic reactions and inflammation. Pitta ailments stem from an excess of heat and acid, and they include poor digestion, heartburn, allergies, acne, hyperacidity (excessive gastric juices), rashes, hives, high blood pressure, dehydration, rosacea, and liver disease. Because pitta governs digestion, regular eating is important to maintain balance. When hun-gry, pittas become hotheaded, cranky, and irritable.

Those with strong pitta tend to be ambitious, competitive, well organized, and task-oriented. Because fire represents transformation, pittas easily absorb information, making them highly intelligent and conspicuous achievers. They are naturally charismatic, eloquent, self-confident, and passionate—all traits our society admires and rewards. Well-balanced pittas make great business and political leaders.

Excess pitta causes these fiery, type A personalities to become opin-ionated, impatient, egotistical, uncompromising, and highly demand-ing. But taking the ayurvedic view, we can better understand that pitta-predominant people are not difficult; it is simply their nature to be the way they are. We can then appreciate their tendencies, avoid being hurt by their actions, and accept them with love.

Vata: Air

The vata dosha embodies air. Vata energy is mobile, dry, rough, and light. Above all, vata governs movement. The nervous system is ruled by ever-changing vata, often making vata-predominant people seem more spirit than matter. Their willowy bodies are light and ethereal. Their skin is dry and thin, rough, and prone to fine lines. Their nails are dry and brittle, and their hair is dry, fine, and often curly. Along with their elongated silhouettes, vatas have thin, chiseled features—sculpted cheekbones, long noses, and thin lips.

Vata disorders mostly relate to the nervous system, manifesting in such problems as paranoia, anxiety, worry, and attention deficit disorder. Vatas' sensory organs are acute, so they need harmonious surroundings; they are easily disturbed by loud or jarring noises, crude images, rough objects, and environmental chaos. They are also prone to kidney disease, bladder problems, low energy, and excessive dryness throughout the skin and body.

The vata personality is creative and excitable. Those dominated by this dosha are forward-looking, open-minded, and flexible. They are early adopters who love innovation and new ideas, and they deeply appreciate beauty in design and art. Vatas love to learn but often feel inadequate, unqualified, and unsure of their abilities despite their knowledge. Socially, they are adaptable and welcoming with excellent interpersonal skills. They also tend to be cerebral, always on the go, changeable, and unpredictable, making them both exciting and frustrating.

When in balance, vatas are charming creatures, artistic, spiritual, and entrepreneurial. When out of balance, they become paranoid, insecure, anxious, hyper, inconsistent, indecisive, and in need of constant reassurance. Long-term vata excess can make vata-dominant people unreliable, rash, impulsive, and frenzied.

Physically, delicate vatas, with their slim, graceful physiques and youthful energy, are today's poster children of ideal beauty. But their true radiance is in their spirituality and optimism.

The ayurvedic mind-body questionnaire will help you determine your dosha. When answering each question, circle the corresponding characteristics that best describe your physical body, behavior, and attitude. Circle all the answers that apply to you, and if none of them apply, simply leave that question blank. Answers should be based on your general tendencies. For example, if you have always had thick, oily hair but it is now becoming dry and is falling out, then choose the "thick and oily" answer because this is how your hair generally is when you are in optimal health. Keep in mind that this is a guide. For the most accurate reading, it is best to consult an ayurvedic doctor or practitioner.

AYURVEDIC MIND–BODY CONSTITUTION QUESTIONNAIRE

What type of weather are you sensitive to?
   A. Dry, cold, and windy
   B. Hot and sunny
   C. Cold and damp

Which characteristics best describe your skin
   A. Dry, thin, and rough
   B. Combination skin, sensitive, hyperpigmentation
   C. Oily, moist, thick

How do your pores look?
   A. Small
   B. Large in T-zone only
   C. Large

Which characteristics best describe your facial complexion?
   A. Fine lines, sallow
   B. Redness, broken capillaries, moles, freckles, rosacea
   C. Blackheads, excess oiliness, soft, youthful, clear

Do you struggle with any of the following skin ailments? (Select all that apply.)
- A. Dehydration
- B. Inflammation
- C. Dullness

- A. Excessive dryness
- B. Rosacea
- C. Swelling from water retention

- A. Dry eczema
- B. Burning eczema
- C. Weepy/itchy eczema

- A. Psoriasis
- B. Rash, hives
- C. Loss of tone/jowls

- A. Cracked skin
- B. Infected blemishes
- C. Cystic acne

- A. Under-eye circles
- B. Contact dermatitis

Which traits describe your facial features? (Select all that apply.)
- A. Chiseled, fine, long, oval
- B. Medium proportions of bone structure
- C. Large bones, round or square

- A. Undefined eyes
- B. Sharp, piercing eyes
- C. Large eyes

- A. Thin, dry lips
- B. Medium lips
- C. Full, soft lips

What type of hair do you have?
- A. Dry, thin, coarse, curly, wiry
- B. Red tones, straight, prematurely gray or balding
- C. Thick, oily, wavy, abundant

What type of fingernails do you have?
- A. Dry, weak, brittle, discolored, irregularly shaped
- B. Soft, medium, pink nail bed
- C. Strong, smooth, regular shaped cuticles

Which description fits your physical build?
- A. Thin, tall, long-limbed
- B. Average height and weight, good muscle tone
- C. Voluptuous, prone to weight gain

Which description fits your physical ability?
- A. Active, quick, poor endurance
- B. Athletic, average strength, intolerant to heat
- C. Lethargic, slow to start, good endurance

What style best describes your thought and learning style?

A. Restless, erratic, creative, chaotic
B. Focused, goal driven
C. Slow learner

A. Quick to learn, poor memory
B. Strong memory
C. Good memory

What is your temperament like?

A. Insecure, unpredictable, and excitable
B. Aggressive, irritable, and impatient
C. Calm, sentimental, and prone to depression

What are your dietary tendencies?

A. Either indulges or follows a strict diet
B. Loves protein, caffeine, and spicy and salty foods
C. Loves sweets, dairy, and carbohydrates

Do you have any of these physical ailments?

A. Kidney problems
B. Hyperacidity, gastric reflux
C. Sinus congestion

A. Constipation
B. Liver disease
C. Asthma

A. Bloating/gas
B. Hypertension
C. Bronchitis

A. Arthritis
B. Inflammatory diseases
C. Obesity

A. Weight loss
B. Hemorrhoids
C. High cholesterol

A. Weak appetite
C. Drowsiness

For women, which best describes your menses?

A. Irregular cycle, scanty flow, severe cramps
B. Heavy bleeding
C. Water retention, slight cramps

Which best describes your gums?

A. Receding
B. Inflamed
C. Thick

Which best describes the state of you joints?

A. Painful, stiff, creaky, unsteady
B. Hot or burning
C. Aching, swollen, retaining fluid

What is your decision-making style?
- A. Creative thinker
- B. Organized thinker
- C. Conservative thinker

What is your work style?
- A. Restless, likes to be busy
- B. Aggressive, likes competition
- C. Calm, likes to relax

How do you approach change?
- A. Seeks change
- B. Plans and proceeds in an organized fashion
- C. Resists change, likes simplicity

Which best describes your social life and relationships within it?
- A. Very social
- B. Very selective
- C. Few friends, but all close

- A. Knows a lot of people
- B. Needs attention
- C. Loyal

- A. Few close friends
- B. Makes enemies easily
- C. Sentimental

Which best describes your spending habits?
- A. Spends impulsively
- B. Spends to achieve a purpose
- C. Likes to save

- B. Spends on luxury goods
- C. Spends reluctantly

Which best describes your role when working on a project?
- A. Conceptualizes
- B. Executes
- C. Maintains

Which qualities best describe your attitudes and behaviors?
- A. Fearful
- B. Angry
- C. Depressive

- A. Nervous
- B. Judgmental
- C. Apathetic

- A. Anxious
- B. Impatient
- C. Patient

- A. Noncommittal
- B. Controlling
- C. Self-indulgent

- A. Youthful
- B. Opinionated
- C. Nurturing

- A. Flexible
- B. Organized
- C. Inflexible

- A. Receptive
- B. Values Equality
- C. Resists giving opinions

- B. Brave

What is your conflict-resolution style?
  A. Accommodating
  B. Insistent
  C. Passive

Total the number of responses in the A, B, and C columns. Mostly A = vata, Mostly B = pitta, Mostly C = kapha

Ayurveda and Contingency

The concept of contingency is fundamental to ayurveda, because the skin (and the whole body) undergoes and is exposed to constant change. The environment exerts many different influences on us, but we must remain balanced in spite of this. When external contingencies occur, we must counteract them with the appropriate dosha-balancing methods that will be discussed in this section. According to ayurveda, these methods are how we maintain well-being. I have often heard ayurvedic doctors say that staying balanced in daily life is like swimming in the ocean; even though the currents may be strong and overpowering, we must stay afloat. We stay balanced by making optimal diet and lifestyle choices. And while understanding our original constitution is important, it is just as important to know what external forces knock us off balance. This introduces another key concept in ayurveda: *prakruti* versus *vikruti*.

Prakruti is our original doshic composition. We are born with perfect health and our special ratio of vata to pitta to kapha. As we move through our lives, we pick up different habits, are exposed to different environments and climates, and choose our behaviors and eating patterns. These choices can either help balance us against environmental influences or create imbalances as we slowly accumulate too much or too little of each dosha. This deviation from prakruti is called vikruti. It is another version of nature versus nurture, or genetics versus environment. For example, someone who works long hours and is constantly sleep deprived will begin to gather more vata in his or her system. Over time, this will create an excess of vata, and this individual will start to exhibit traits of vata imbalance. He or she may lose muscle mass, and feel scattered and insecure; and his or her skin may begin to dehydrate and thin. If this goes unresolved, this may worsen and translate into a full blown vata dysfunction, causing kidney disease, kidney stones, or anxiety disorders.

Everyone has a natural inclination to accumulate the same type of energy as that of their prakruti's predominant dosha and is attracted to environments that increase that energy. For example, those with strong kapha are prone to lethargy, fostering even more kapha; those with strong pitta are prone to inflammation and perfectionism, leading to more pitta; and those with strong vata love change and irregular schedules, promoting more vata. But you can use this knowledge to empower yourself. When you are confronted by environments and external factors that might throw you off balance, you can make appropriate choices to help maintain your energetic harmony, optimal health, and vital beauty.

WEATHER CONTINGENCIES

The weather has doshic qualities that can cause changes within the body. It is a strong influence because it is inescapable. Being very sensitive to weather, I find myself feeling irritable in the heat because of my pitta dominance. Pitta weather is warm and sunny, and the fire dosha increases when the temperature gets hotter, giving fiery pitta individuals rashes, hives, inflammation, and breakouts. They can also exhibit pitta's emotional characteristics, such as becoming short-tempered and easily agitated. Those with strong pitta must balance a hot environment by eating raw, cooling foods; avoiding exercises that overheat the body; and opting for soothing activities such as yoga and swimming. Pittas feel most calm in cool weather.

Damp and cold is kapha weather. Those with high kapha feel lethargic, heavy, and puffy from water retention in this type of environment. They may also experience swollen eyes and excessive mucus. To counter this, kaphas should eat stimulating, warm foods and practice exercises that promote circulation. Waking up early also helps reduce kapha in this type of weather. Kapha accumulates in the winter when it is wet or snowy, and it is expressed in the spring with the rainy season. Kaphas are most in balance in hot, dry climates.

Windy, crisp weather promotes vata. In this environment, vata types feel scattered, anxious, and forgetful. This usually occurs in the fall, which is also a time of transition. Because vata governs change, the changeover from summer to winter is a time for insomnia as well as dehydrated skin. The best way to balance this is by keeping the body hydrated and warm. Eating nourishing, dense foods and moisturizing the skin with sesame oil will pacify vata energy. Vatas function best when the weather is warm and humid.

DIET CONTINGENCIES

Because food is our fuel, diet may be one of the most effective ways to balance the body. Like weather influences, food also has doshic qualities. Below is a chart outlining food that shares energetic properties. It shows what must be avoided in order to prevent doshic excess, and what foods have balancing energetic properties.

When trying to reduce pitta and inflammation, avoid hot, spicy, sour, and acidic foods. How food is prepared is also important, as pittas must also stay away from overcooked, fried, and barbecued foods due to their excess heat. This is essential, especially when skin problems flare up.

When trying to pacify kapha, avoid heavy, creamy, fatty foods that are also sweet, salty, or tart. An "antikapha" diet is instrumental if you are trying to lose weight.

When trying to manage the vata constitution, avoid dry, crunchy, and astringent foods. Foods like crackers, fat-free products, dry meat, and vegetables in the cabbage family are all hard to digest and cause excess gas and constipation in delicate vata systems.

As we will discuss in the next section, it is not only what you eat, it is also when you eat that gives the body and skin the best chance of absorbing the nutrients to repair and protect themselves.

TIME CONTINGENCIES

We respond to all three doshas during the course of the day, because different doshic elements increase at different hours. This gives us clues as to the optimal time to eat, take medicinal herbs, and rest.

Kapha energy is highest from 6 A.M. to 10 A.M. and from 6 P.M. to 10 P.M. One of the best ways to decrease kapha is to get up before 6 A.M. to ensure that you are active and stimulated during kapha hours, shaking out the heavy earth and water energy from your body. This is also why you actually feel drowsy when you sleep past 10 A.M., as you pick up and foster more of this energy. Conversely, you should go to bed during the evening kapha hours, because it is easiest to fall asleep when kapha is strong.

If you feel sleepy and are ready to go to bed but stay up past kapha hours, you may experience a "second wind." This is because you have moved into pitta time. Pitta is strongest from 10 A.M. to 2 P.M. and from 10 P.M. to 2 A.M. Your largest meal should be lunch, eaten before 2 P.M. while pitta is ignited and aids digestion.

Vata time is from 2 A.M. to 6 A.M. and from 2 P.M. to 6 P.M.; it is strongest during hours of transition (dawn and dusk). This is why many

Ayurvedic Food Chart

	Vata		Pitta		Kapha	
	EAT	AVOID	EAT	AVOID	EAT	AVOID
Vegetables	Beets Carrots Radishes String beans Zucchini	Bell peppers Broccoli Brussels sprouts Cabbage Cauliflower Raw vegetables	Alfalfa, pea, and bean sprouts Asparagus Broccoli Celery Cucumbers Leafy greens	Eggplant Hot peppers Radishes Tomatoes	Asparagus Beets Bell peppers Broccoli Leafy greens Onions	Cucumbers Zucchini
Starches	Cooked oats Rice Sweet potatoes Wheat	Barley Buckwheat Corn Dry oats Potatoes (all except sweet potatoes) Rye	Barley Cooked oats Potatoes (all) Rice (basmati) Wheat	Buckwheat Corn Dry oats Millet Rice (brown) Rye	Barley Corn Dry oats Millet Rye	All potatoes Cooked oats Rice Wheat
Proteins	All nuts All seeds Beef Chicken (white meat) Duck Eggs Seafood	All legumes (except mung beans, tofu, and black and red lentils) Lamb Pork	All legumes (except lentils) Chicken (white meat) Egg whites Turkey (white meat)	All nuts All seeds (except sunflower and pumpkin) Beef Egg yolks Lamb Pork Seafood	All legumes (except kidney beans, soy, black lentils, and mung beans) Chicken (dark meat) Freshwater fish Shrimp	All nuts All seeds (except sunflower and pumpkin) Beef Lamb Pork Saltwater fish
Fruits	Avocados Bananas Berries Grapes Lemons Melons	Apples Dried fruits Pears	Apples Avocados Mango Melons Pears	Grapefruit Lemons Oranges (sour) Peaches Plums (sour)	Apples Berries Peaches Pears Prunes	All high-sugar, tropical fruits Avocados Bananas Melons Pineapple
Fats	All dairy All oils (especially sesame oil)		Coconut oil Ghee Milk Olive oil Sunflower oil	Almond oil Cheese Corn oil Safflower oil Sour cream Yogurt	Almond, flax, and sunflower oil (in small amounts) Goat's milk and ghee (in small amounts)	All dairy All oils
Other	All spices (especially hot, warming spices) All sweeteners	Caffeine	All sweeteners (except honey and molasses) Cooling spices (parsley, mint, turmeric, fennel, coriander)	Caffeine Hot spices Salt	All spices (except salt) Raw honey	All sweeteners (except honey) Salt

people suffer from insomnia if they do not go to bed early enough, as vata is awakened in the body during the late hours. One of the best ways to combat insomnia is to go to bed during kapha times of day. Ayurveda also says to eat your last meal before 6 P.M. or sundown, during vata time. Avoid eating during kapha time when metabolic function is slow.

When trying to cleanse or remove excess dosha, it is best to take the dosha-balancing herbal remedy at the time of day when that specific dosha is strongest. For example, taking Trikatu early in the morning during Kapha time will intensely clear kapha. This way, the body accumulates as much of that energy as possible so it can be eliminated. See the sidebar on page 58 for more information.

MENSTRUAL CYCLE CONTINGENCIES

Menses affect women's moods, complexions, and food preferences, because the doshas fluctuate throughout the menstrual cycle.

Kapha is high between the end of the menstrual flow and the next ovulation, and this fertile, maternal energy prepares the womb. This is when many women often experience puffiness and water retention.

Pitta is high from ovulation until flow begins. Those with excess pitta can experience inflammatory premenstrual syndrome (PMS).

Vata is high during the actual days of flow, because vata governs movement. According to ayurveda, the loss of blood equates to a loss of vitality. Rest and pampering are advisable during the first two days of menstrual flow.

EMOTIONAL CONTINGENCIES

How we think and feel impacts our body more than most of us realize. Because the doshas govern different emotions, an imbalance in any of them wreaks havoc on our emotional well-being. The opposite is also true. When we experience emotional disruption, this affects the state of the doshas within us.

Feeling anxious or insecure increases vata. Conversely, when there is an excess of vata, we feel less sure of ourselves and less grounded. The root of vata emotions is fear, and the more fear we experience, the more vata we will acquire.

Excess pitta emotion comes out as anger and manipulation. Pitta governs the ego, and while we need ego to survive, excess egotism and aggression are signs of a pitta excess. These characteristics are often fostered by a pitta's perfectionism as well as self-pressure.

When in balance, kapha makes us compassionate, calm, and nurturing, but when there is too much kapha energy, we become needy and feel hopeless and depressed. The heavier our emotional state, the more kapha we accumulate. We may sometimes have the strength and discipline to lift our own spirits; at other times, we need the help of a kapha-pacifying diet and lifestyle to overcome these feelings.

In some ways, emotional factors are the hardest to treat and change because our attachment to personal behaviors and patterns is strong. They often require a shift in perspective, not simply habit. But in other ways, they are easy to change because once you identify the doshic issue, it is within your power to resolve it.

STAGE-OF-LIFE CONTINGENCIES

Each dosha is tied to a specific stage of life. Kapha is strongest in youth, pitta prevails in middle age, and vata becomes the dominating influence in maturity and old age.

Stage-of-life contingencies can make self-diagnosis difficult. When I discovered ayurveda in my midteens, I thought I was a pitta-kapha, because I displayed many kapha characteristics. I was lethargic; had an intolerance to wet, mucus-forming foods (such as milk and heavy starches); and was hesitant about change. When I was properly di-agnosed by an ayurvedic doctor, I was surprised to find that I was a pitta-vata. My kapha afflictions were partly due to an imbalance in that dosha that was emphasized because I was in the kapha stage of life. One way to differentiate between your prakruti and your vikruti, which is influenced by your stage of life, is to ask yourself if you have always had the traits you recognize now. When in doubt, consult an ayurvedic doctor, who can easily determine the difference by reading your pulse.

Kapha is strongest during the formative years, from birth through puberty and into the early twenties. This is when people grow physi-cally and accumulate knowledge. They have baby fat, and their skin is as moist as it will ever be. They are prone to self-centeredness and self-indulgence, and memory is at its best.

This is also the time when many children experience weepy eczema and excessive mucus from allergies; teens tend to have acne pustules. Avoiding moist, kapha-promoting foods (dairy products, sweet and salty foods, starches) helps to alleviate these ailments.

Kaphas also love to sleep in, which aggravates their problems, so rising early helps mitigate such problems. Cardiovascular exercise is also recommended, since stimulation is the key to clearing excess ka-pha. Ayurveda prescribes a vigorous massage, using powder instead of oil, to promote circulation. Through the traction of the powder, fatty tissue is mobilized, and kapha stagnation is dispersed.

The twenties through the forties are the pitta years. This is when life is action-oriented and career focused. Excess pitta is caused by overambitious expectations and by pushing the body too hard. This sometimes leads to a compromised liver and food sensitivities. It is also the time when rosacea (known as adult acne), along with broken capil-laries and uneven pigmentation, is most likely to occur.

Avoiding hot, overcooked, spicy foods helps soothe pitta excesses, as do cooler environmental temperatures. Unfortunately, pittas love strenuous exercise, which creates more heat. Yogic practices and meditation help balance out the body's fire, and they calm and clear the mind. Pitta skin cannot handle heavy oils because they increase heat, but lightweight oils such as coconut and jojoba are great for cooling the skin. Saunas and hot tubs should be avoided.

Vata becomes influential as people move into maturity. They grow more spiritual in their later years, but though they may have gained in wisdom, they have likely decreased in matter. A decline in collagen production triggers a loss in weight and height as well. The skin becomes drier, wrinkled, and thinner. Thoughts may become more erratic, like air, while memories are difficult to grasp.

Promoting kapha is beneficial as a countermeasure, and those with strong kapha seem to age the best. Eating moist, heavy foods and getting ample sleep is beneficial in minimizing vata excess, as is daily body and scalp massage with sesame oil. Vatas, in particular, should have regular, relaxing massages with heavy, nourishing oils. Absorbing such oils through the skin pacifies vata and counters an overactive nervous system.

While kapha combats aging caused by an excess of pitta and vata, it is said that pitta and vata doshas are the action-created energies that allow the soul to ascend to the next realm. Each dosha has its role and is part of our natural life cycle. Though our youth-obsessed culture encourages us to fight the aging process, beauty can also come from letting nature take its course.

Ayurveda and Holistic Beauty

While I was in India, I was astonished by how much beauty was integrated into the culture. Even in poor or polluted communities, people still found ways of surrounding themselves with lovely things. They decorated their cars and trucks with bright, fresh-flower garlands bought from street vendors, bringing color to grimy streets. I loved how people used real flowers, despite their fragility, to bring wonderful aromas to the surroundings.

Beauty is an inherent part of ayurvedic philosophy. From daily self-massage and grooming rituals to using the skin as a diagnostic tool, this ideology has an innate appreciation for the importance of beauty and self-care. Many healing practices are specifically aimed at maintaining beauty, and treatments for acne and other skin problems are even outlined in ayurveda's oldest scriptures.

But it is important to understand that attractiveness for the sake of vanity is not valued; rather, beauty is an indication that the body and doshas are in balance. Minor skin issues can be early warning signs of internal imbalances that may lead to disease if left untreated. When we look at the ayurvedic view of how disease manifests, we understand how beauty practices are part of illness prevention as well as a significant component of maintaining proper doshic balance. When one or more doshic energies accumulate to excess, they begin to implant and disperse themselves throughout the body; according to ayurveda, this causes skin problems and other more serious ailments.

THE SIX STAGES OF DISEASE (SAMPRAPTI)

From an ayurvedic perspective, disease is not something with which we are randomly afflicted; rather, it is a process. At the root of disease is an imbalance caused by excess dosha energy. Once we understand this, the importance of monitoring our doshas becomes clear.

Dr. Vasant Lad compares the disease process to a leaky faucet filling a bucket with water. When the water overflows, it spills into your garden, soaking the soil and giving life to sprouting weeds of illness.

In this situation, the faucet comprises lifestyle habits that create excess dosha (the water), and when it spills beyond your prakruti, this out-of-balance doshic energy scavenges your tissues. When it finds a place to settle, it expresses itself as disease. This poetic description of the development and course of illness shows that there are many components to becoming sick, so if you are proactive and listen to your body, you have many opportunities to prevent it.

The rest of this section outlines the six stages of illness according to ayurvedic philosophy.

Stage One: Accumulation (Sanchaya). In the first stage of disease, one or more doshas begin to accumulate. This is usually due to improper diet or lifestyle, one that does not resonate with our natural prakruti. Early imbalances and symptoms at this stage occur only in the gastrointestinal tract. Each dosha corresponds to an organ of digestion, so when kapha, pitta, or vata accumulates, subtle imbalances occur in the associated organ. The seat of kapha is in the stomach, so when kapha builds up, we may feel heaviness or fullness there. Pitta is based in the small intestine, so an excess of pitta collects there and may cause a sensation of heat around the belly button. Vata is associated with the colon, so when this energy increases, we may feel constipated, bloated, or uncomfortable in that area.

During this stage, we are still healthy, and the body attempts to heal by itself. We crave foods that will help us rebalance, so following these impulses is integral to staying healthy.

Stage Two: Provocation (Prakopa). The second stage is when the doshic accumulation steadily increases (the bucket becomes fuller). This happens when we have ignored the accumulation stage and have continued to live, eat, and behave in ways that aggravate one or more of our doshas. The imbalance is still contained in the gastrointestinal tract, but symptoms become more acute, and we experience regular discomfort. At this stage, we can still easily restore ourselves to optimum health through dietary choices and other simple remedies, but if the problem is not addressed, it becomes much more difficult to reverse.

Stage Three: Dispersion (Prasara). It is at this stage that excess dosha spreads to other parts of the body. Instead of our tastes and cravings calling for substances and activities that would help to reharmonize the doshas, our impulses now shift toward choices that further aggravate the imbalance. This helps the overflowing dosha gather energy and continue moving. This is the stage when dosha energy travels to secondary sites in the body, often affecting the skin. While pitta may manifest as hives or a rash, vata displays itself through dehydrated skin. Kapha travels into the lymphatic system, causing puffiness and water retention.

Stage Four: Deposition (Sthana Samsraya). The fourth stage is the point at which the overflow is deposited in a weak spot in the body—most likely, a place that has suffered trauma or injury in the past or has low resistance. Excess dosha does not settle where tissues and tissue metabolism are strong, but it flourishes in compromised areas. This is why it is so important to keep our immune system and tissues healthy and to pay special attention to rehabilitation after trauma or surgery.

Stage Five: Manifestation (Vyatkti). During this stage, the disease develops further. The qualities of each dosha are amplified in the weak spot. Vata dryness or depletion (i.e. dehydration, weakness, low energy) will occur with vata imbalances; pitta inflammation will appear; and kapha dampness and stagnation (i.e. mucous, lack of action) will affect the point of manifestation. The function of the affected tissue or organ is impeded, and it is important to seek guidance from an experienced holistic practitioner. This is usually the point at which disease is identified in Western medicine.

Stage Six: Differentiation/Destruction (Bheda). At this last stage, the disease is fully established, and it begins to affect surrounding tissues and organs. Structural changes begin to take place in the tissue, and the function of the newly affected body parts becomes impaired.

One example of a sixth-stage beauty ailment is psoriasis. In its earlier stages, the skin is dry and irritated; later on, this autoimmune disorder starts to affect other parts of the body (as in psoriasis-related arthritis), inhibits temperature regulation through the skin, and requires intensive treatment that may include hospitalization and steroid injections.

Another skin-related disorder, rosacea, at first causes dilated capillaries but can eventually change the texture and structure of the skin, resulting in deformation. This severe form of the disease often occurs in individuals with a history of alcohol abuse. They accumulate so much pitta from the heat-inducing quality of alcohol that the ailment moves from the blood system to the skin, causing facial deformity. This occurs most often in the area of the nose, which in ayurveda is related to the heart (also governed by pitta).

Face Mapping

Examining your skin is a wonderful way to identify the state of your overall health. While facial blemishes and wrinkles may appear unsightly, they can actually help you monitor possible internal problems. Dermatologists and beauty consultants often simply prescribe harsh creams to camouflage these skin imperfections, whereas ayurvedic practitioners use them as a guide to "read" the internal organs. This reading is called face mapping.

In ayurveda, each dosha governs different sections of the face, organs, and limbs. While this makes for a very complex ideology, it provides a simple guide for diagnosis. As shown in the first face map, vata governs the top of the face from the eyes to the hairline, pitta governs the middle section between the eyes and the mouth, and kapha governs the lower face. Skin ailments in each of these areas are often due to an imbalance of the corresponding dosha.

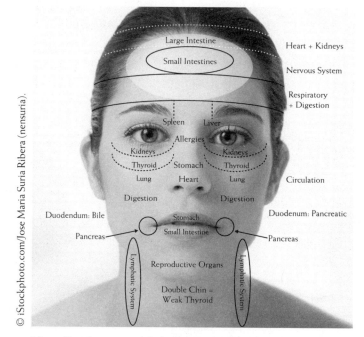

Note: Facial areas are labeled as in a mirror image.

The forehead, which is the thinnest and driest area of the face, is where vata expresses itself. Worry lines are caused by vata emotions such as anxiety and fear, which also result in insomnia and other stress-rela0ted disorders that deepen these lines further. Many people experience pore-congestion isolated to the forehead, which is often linked to constipation, as the colon is also governed by vata. When treating vatas for dry skin, it is also necessary to detoxify the colon and calm the mind.

Pitta rules the center of the face, where rosacea, whiteheads, and broken capillaries are often found. According to ayurveda, rosacea is a cardiovascular disorder caused by anger, jealousy, and stress resulting from pressure to succeed (this usually is self-inflicted, since pittas are highly ambitious).

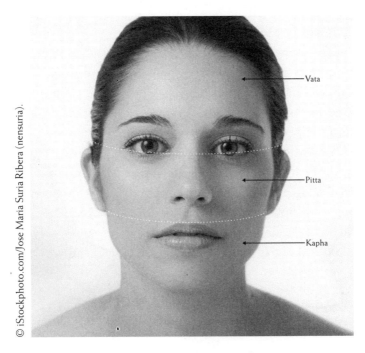

© iStockphoto.com/Jose Maria Suria Ribera (nensuria).

Teenagers often have red, blistered acne in this area caused by the hormonal heat of puberty. Acne restricted to the cheeks or nose should be treated with cooling herbs, blood purification, and detoxification of the small intestine. Smoking also increases internal heat. Smoking cessation helps lessen both the signs of rosacea and irritated breakouts in this section of the face.

The lower face is governed by kapha. Cystic acne, with kapha qualities of fluid retention and swelling, is most commonly found on the chin and along the jawline. These types of deep-seated blemishes are also caused by hormonal imbalances. The kapha area often breaks out in cysts because of internal toxin retention and stagnation of lymphatic fluid. It can also reflect lethargy, emotional repression, or an inability to let go. An imbalance here may manifest as a double chin (excess fat) caused by hypothyroidism.

Acne in the kapha region should be treated with lymphatic stimulation through massage and exercise and a kapha-reducing diet low in sweets, salt, and oily and fatty foods.

As noted in the preceding discussion, your complexion also gives insight into the health of your internal organs. In ayurveda—as in the systems of reflexology and acupuncture—these organs relate to specific parts of the face and body, as shown on the second face map. It is fascinating to learn about how ancient practitioners discovered these interactions and how external imperfections reflect what is going on inside the body. Again, this demonstrates that no skin problem can be totally cured without addressing lifestyle and total health.

Health, Beauty, and the Internal Organs

When you discover the root cause of your imbalances, you are able to address and treat organ dysfunctions through truly effective, long-term beauty care. The following sections outline how the internal organs are related to health and beauty issues in ayurvedic terms.

LIVER

Making sure your liver is functional and healthy is essential for a clear complexion. The liver is the body's filtration system and is central to the elimination of waste. It also plays a role in regulating the hormones. When your bowels do not function properly, waste saturates the liver and impairs its function as well. It becomes like a wet sponge that cannot absorb or filter anything. Toxins spill over to other organs and are purged through the skin (through irritation and blemishes) or the lungs (by coughing up mucus). Toxins spilling over into other organs and impaired bowel function are related to filtering hormones and are governed by pitta (the source of inflammation).

Frown lines between the eyebrows are due to an overheated liver and a dysfunctional spleen. The wrinkles perpendicular to the right brow relate to the liver, and those to the left relate to the spleen, so cleansing both organs is an excellent antiaging practice. Treating frown lines superficially with Botox injections simply adds toxins to the body and further exhausts the liver.

To detoxify the liver, start gently by eating leafy greens supplemented with a milk thistle tincture. Bitters reduce excess pitta making milk thistle, dandelion, and neem herbs ideal for purging the liver and mitigating internal fire. (See the sidebar on page 58 for more information on specific herbs.)

KIDNEYS

Caring for the kidneys is an important beauty practice, especially if you want to minimize signs of aging. Weak kidneys cause undereye circles. If the kidneys are taxed, this also interferes with sleep and contributes further to those dark circles. Because the kidneys regulate water metabolism, improper function can result in puffiness under the eyes as well as generalized body edema (water retention).

The kidneys, which also help sustain the bones and hair and are governed by vata, weaken with age. This is why hair loss, osteoporosis, and arthritis are linked to aging. Stress also has a negative effect on the kidneys and thus plays a major role in balding.

When the kidneys are overworked, vata is aggravated. This results in anxiety, fear, and worry. It also leads to dry skin. Strengthening the kidneys involves decreasing salt intake, drinking plenty of water, limiting protein consumption, and getting a proper amount of rest. Pacifying vata through a daily self-massage with sesame oil and taking vata-reducing herbs like ashwagandha and shatavari also helps restore balance to the kidneys.

STOMACH

The stomach is a kapha organ and where this energy accumulates, but its digestive function is dictated by stomach *agni* (fire). This digestive fire, whether strong or weak, is closely related to pitta. Symptoms of high pitta include acid stomach, heartburn, and stomach ulcers, often paired with skin inflammation.

The stomach corresponds to the upper lip (the lower lip corresponds to the small intestine). When the stomach is dehydrated, it is expressed through dry lips. Treating this condition involves hydrating the gastrointestinal tract by eating easily digestible, water-rich foods such as most squash, crunchy string beans, and fresh berries.

SMALL INTESTINE

The small intestine is a pitta organ, and when it is out of balance, it contributes to skin inflammation. People with rosacea, rashes, or a tendency to allergic reactions in the facial area often experience energy pushing upward from this major pitta site.

Excess heat in the small intestine also causes dryness in the body and contributes to dryness of the lower lip. This usually indicates dehydration in the gastrointestinal tract in general. In such cases, applying lip balm is not sufficient; cleansing and hydrating the small intestine is required.

The small intestine is also the site where nutrients are absorbed.

When it does not function properly, energy levels decrease and skin is devitalized due to malabsorption.

Amalaki is an excellent herb for eliminating heat and clearing pitta congestion in the small intestine through purging. A mild laxative, amalaki is one of the three ingredients that make up the tridoshic staple cleansing formula Triphala. It is the pitta balancing component of Triphala, and also addresses pitta vitiation throughout the body. Drinking aloe vera juice is also a good way to clean the small intestine. This gentle laxative reduces internal inflammation and helps to rehydrate the digestive system.

COLON

Ensuring the regularity and comfort of the colon is one of the most important things you can do to promote beautiful skin. The bowels are the first avenue of elimination, and they must be cleansed before any other organ. While it is also important to cleanse the liver, kidneys, gallbladder, and so on, if the bowels are backed up, other detoxification is impossible. This contributes to blemishes and skin dehydration.

While they may feel they eliminate regularly, many people do not realize that they should ideally have bowel movements twice a day. If waste is not purged from the body, toxins accumulate, causing illness and dehydration.

Because the colon is a vata organ, when the large intestine is not functioning properly, breakouts and black heads appear in the vata area of the face: the forehead. To treat this, it is important to understand that nourishment and moisture help keep it healthy and balanced. Hydration and an increase in water and oil consumption pacify vata and ensure that no dry stool is left in the intestines (further drying out the body). Colonics and enemas are helpful for this purpose. Colonics, or colon irrigation, involve inserting water into the colon through the anus to alleviate constipation, but ayurveda advocates medicated enemas (called *bastis*), which are said to be less abrasive. Bastis can use oils or herbal infusions to loosen dry stool while healing the intestinal wall.

I have seen many types of health benefits result from these therapies, but it is important to avoid overstimulating the colon. If you decide to engage in colonic irrigation or regular enemas, have a qualified practitioner outline a series of treatments that is tailored to your individual needs. Overwashing the colon can be irritating, increase vata, and damage the intestinal wall.

Laxatives are another means of colon upkeep, but one of the principles of ayurveda is that no food or therapy is universally good. Each person and each dosha responds to different things. For instance, vatas are so dry that psyllium (a natural laxative) constipates them, whereas kaphas have enough moisture for it to be effective. Vatas do better with moist laxatives such as soaked prunes, mangoes, and castor oil; kaphas need roughage and fiber. Pittas respond well to cooling laxatives such as aloe vera juice, rhubarb, and senna; they can also use castor oil. If you are concerned or confused by different laxatives, Triphala is a traditional tridoshic blend for regular elimination.

REPRODUCTIVE ORGANS

According to ayurveda, the reproductive organs are important because they create and maintain much of our *ojas*, which is the fluid or sap of life energy. This is why virility is considered to be related to overall vitality, and abstinence is recommended when the immune system is low. Vertical wrinkles on the upper lip are caused by weakness in the reproductive organs, such as sterility and sexual debility. Chainsmokers tend to develop wrinkles here because cigarette smoking can damage the sex organs.

Ayurveda prescribes shatavari (the term literally means "woman who possesses one hundred husbands") to cleanse and regenerate these organs. It is used to increase fertility in both men and women, address menstrual issues, and support the transition of menopause.

HEART

Excess redness in the skin and broken capillaries on the nose signify an overworked heart and high blood pressure. The heart is a pitta organ and is closely connected to the circulatory system, which is also governed by pitta (specifically the red blood cells). The heart is in charge of the capillaries. Alcoholics often acquire facial redness and broken capillaries, most often in the nose area, because alcohol increases heat and pitta.

The heart is also considered to be part of the mind, and emotional health registers on the face, specifically the nose. When you are stressed or weighed down emotionally, your heart is taxed, affecting your complexion. As mentioned earlier, rosacea is a perfect example of how the heart affects the skin.

Cleansing the blood and strengthening the heart are important. Neem and burdock root, as well as rose tonics, are three natural remedies that help heal the heart.

LUNGS

The health of the lungs is reflected in the skin and body hair, which receive nourishment and water passed to them by these kapha organs. When the lungs are taxed with allergies and respiratory problems, they cannot disperse fluid, which makes the skin and the hair dry and brittle. The lungs are related to the cheek area so dryness, breakouts, or irritation can be found there when the lungs are unhealthy.

The lungs also have an important role in detoxification. The skin, lungs, and colon are all channels of elimination, which is why allergic reactions often occur in these organs as well; the body tries to rid itself of toxicity through redness and inflammation, coughing, or diarrhea. When the lungs are depleted, mucus often accumulates in them. The presence of excess mucus (a form of toxic water/moisture in the body) causes congestion in the sinuses and nasal passages, which can also cause facial puffiness. In such cases, kapha needs to be pacified. Traditional herbal remedies like Trikatu (see the sidebar) mitigate dampness and support digestion for people with high prakruti kapha.

Licorice is another excellent herb for supporting lung health. This, of course, would be taken in its purest form, without sugar or additives. Teas, capsules, or pure powder are best. It rids the lungs of mucus but is also a regenerative supplement and very harmonizing; it is said to be the best traditional lung tonic.

STAPLES OF AYURVEDIC MEDICINE

Here are some of ayurveda's most common natural remedies for supporting the organs and rebalancing the doshas. All of these remedies are available as dried herbs. Unlike vitamins and extracts, which are concentrated and sometimes hard for the body to process, these ayurvedic medicines are closer to being whole foods. Many of them are common spices that can simply be eaten in food. They can all be found at health food stores, in specialty herb shops, or through online retailers (see "Rejuvenating Resources" at the end of this book).

Amalaki: Amalaki pacifies pitta. This tart fruit is also excellent for purging the bowels and supporting digestion. It is a great anti-inflammatory and is packed with antioxidants. One amalaki fruit contains the same amount of vitamin C as twenty oranges.

While its powder is used in Triphala, amalaki can be eaten fresh, although it is difficult to find the fruit outside of Asia.

Ashwagandha: Ashwagandha is one of the best vata-pacifying herbs in ayurveda. This nutritive plant builds muscle, strengthens skin tissue, calms the nervous system, and protects the body against stress. Most often, ashwagandha roots are dried and made into powder, which can then be taken in capsules or by the spoonful. The average dose is approximately a half to a whole teaspoon a day. Ashwagandha can also be infused in oils (used topically in self-massage) and ghees (used in food preparation).

Bibhitaki: Bibhitaki fruit has a heating effect and reduces kapha. It rids the body of impurities and excess mucus, allowing for better absorption of nutrients. Bibhitaki is also used for deep purification; as an antiseptic; and for its antiparasitic, deworming properties.

Guduchi: A rejuvenating remedy (rasayana), guduchi is tridoshic, but it is especially effective in pacifying vata and pitta. It is excellent for antiaging, as it protects tissues, promotes mental clarity, and helps resist infection by enhancing the white blood cells. Guduchi itself is a climbing vine, and an ayurvedic doctor once told me that its rapid growth and resilience reflected its healing properties. It is useful for brightening the skin, because it purifies the blood and cleanses and regenerates the liver. One teaspoon twice a day is a standard dose, but the powder can also be mixed with water to make a paste that is applied topically to clarify the skin.

Haritaki: Haritaki calms vata and is a rich source of amino acids that help to increase energy levels and to build muscle and other tissues. It gently clears the bowels and the body's channels of transportation, improving circulation, the body's nerve communication, and overall health. Haritaki strengthens mental capabilities and promotes astuteness and awareness.

Neem: Neem is a bitter herb that decreases excess pitta and kapha. This remedy is ideal for treating cystic acne (along with other internal cysts and growths), eradicating parasites, and fighting infection because of its anti-inflammatory and dampness-purging properties. Ayurveda uses neem in toothpaste or as a tooth powder, because it soothes sensitive and bleeding gums and kills bacteria. It is also traditionally used for skin ailments, because it purifies the blood matter and the liver.

Neem has a very strong taste, so while the powder can be taken by the half teaspoonful, it is much more palatable in capsule form. The standard dose is one to three capsules with meals. Neem oil is also widely available and is used topically on rashes, itchy skin, bug bites, and inflammation. It can also be applied to the scalp to treat dandruff.

Shatavari: Shatavari root nourishes kapha and reduces pitta and vata. Because it promotes kapha energy, it is an excellent supplement for depletion and wasting diseases, as it boosts the immune system and supports robust tissues. It is also effective for reducing acid and is traditionally used to increase fertility and improve breast milk production. This herb can be taken in capsules or as a powder. It also comes combined with cane sugar as "shatavari grains," which can be added to hot water to make a nourishing drink.

Trikatu: Trikatu is a preparation of three spicy herbs that purges excess kapha and dampness from the body. Composed of dried ginger, pippali, and black pepper, this traditional remedy stimulates the digestive system, breaks down toxins, speeds up metabolic function, and purifies the lungs and respiratory system. Trikatu can be taken in pure powder form in capsules, or sprinkled on food as a spice blend. The normal daily dose is half a teaspoon, or two capsules, taken either before or after meals. When Trikatu is taken before eating, its action kindles and strengthens the digestion; when it is taken after eating, it detoxifies the body.

Triphala: An ancient blend of three dried fruits (amalaki, bibhitaki, and haritaki), Triphala is used for its cleansing and nourishing actions. It is probably ayurveda's most common remedy and is used for general health maintenance and as a gentle daily laxative. Triphala is tridoshic, and each ingredient balances one of the three doshic energies. It comes in powder form and is usually taken nightly (half a teaspoon) with warm water. Triphala is so highly regarded in ayurveda for its nurturing and balancing properties that it is even the basis for an old Indian saying: "No mother? Don't worry, as long as you have Triphala."

Tulsi: Tulsi, also known as holy basil, is a sacred herb and one of the easiest ayurvedic supplements to find. The dried leaves of this plant are made into aromatic teas or pulverized into powders, and they heighten awareness, promote enlightenment, and facilitate breathing. Tulsi grounds vata and clears excess kapha. A study entitled "Evaluation of Hypoglycemic and Antioxidant Effect of Ocimum Sanctum" (tulsi) which was published in the *Indian Journal of Clinical Biochemistry* found that tulsi helped to regulate blood glucose levels because of its antioxidant properties.

Turmeric: Turmeric is one of my favorite herbs. While it is tri-doshic, I use it mostly for soothing pitta, since it is a powerful anti-inflammatory. It is also excellent for treating acne; it cleanses the blood, supports the liver, and has antibacterial properties. Turmeric root powder is common in Asian cooking and can be sprinkled on food or added to curry dishes. I often recommend taking it in capsules, because its yellow color can make a mess, dyeing skin as well as household surfaces and fabrics. I have even used it as a natural self-tanner. When taking capsules, start with two to three pills after meals. Not only does it provide the afore-mentioned benefits, but it also decreases bloating and helps heal digestive issues such as chronic indigestion and inflammation in the GI tract.

It is advisable to consult an ayurvedic practitioner or doctor be-fore using any of these herbs, especially if you are pregnant or nursing. This way, you can be sure that you have the best rem-edies for your constitution and health issues, and that you are taking them in their proper form and dosage. (See "Rejuvenating Resources" at the end of this book for suggestions on finding an ayurvedic health center or professional in your area.)

As you can see, ayurveda outlines beauty as a reflection of well-being within our bodies. When our doshas or internal organs are not in bal-ance, this affects the state of our skin. Now that we understand the basics of ayurveda and its view of self-care, we will discuss the Western view of the skin and learn how we can use both of the methodologies to attain a healthy complexion.

Three

Skin Basics

We usually judge our skin on its esthetic value instead of appreciating it as the body's largest organ. We often abuse it with harsh products and chemical peels or simply by bumping, bruising, scraping, and cutting it without any real awareness of the stress such hurts cause this valuable body shield. Fortunately, the skin has an amazing capacity for self-repair. It is a complex network of capillaries, sweat glands, hair follicles, and tissue cells.

The skin is the body's armor; it protects the muscles, nerves, and internal organs, and it contains all the other systems. It also controls what passes in and out of the body, acting as its gatekeeper. We could not function without this supple, highly resilient barrier.

The skin also emits and disperses heat, thereby regulating body temperature. When we are too hot, the pores open to release heat; this is called vasodilation. When we are cold, the pores close up, trapping body heat; this is called vasoconstriction. Vasoconstriction causes goose bumps, because when the pores tighten, they form bumps and cause the hair to stand on end. According to the naturopath Leon Chaitow, one of the best ways to relax and calm the nervous system is through maintaining a consistent body temperature. For example, soaking in a warm bath relieves stress because body temperature remains the same while you are submerged in the water. This example also shows the connection between mind and body and how emotional grounding and relaxation can be encouraged through working with the skin.

Another function of the skin is, of course, tactile sensation. According to ayurveda, the skin's sensory nerve endings are connected to vata and the central nervous system. Thus, a good massage with vata-pacifying sesame oil helps to harmonize the mind.

The skin is a juncture of our internal, external, and emotional selves. It reflects our emotions: when we are embarrassed, we blush; when we are shocked, we turn pale. Since the skin mirrors the emotions, it is not surprising that skin ailments often have emotional triggers. I know that stress is the main cause of my eczema outbreaks, and many of my rosacea clients say stress causes their flare-ups. One of my clients gets a rash on her elbows every time she takes an exam. Lines on the forehead, dehydration, and acne are also related to anxiety and other forms of emotional distress.

The skin is actually an organ of detoxification through excreting sebum (oil) and sweating. According to ayurveda, perspiration is a form of gentle detoxification and is even part of the preparation for the *panchakarma* process (detoxification through five actions, which is discussed in chapter 8). But many of us prevent this healthy physiological reaction by using pore-clogging products. We actively try to stop sweat production by using antiperspirants. Not only does this inhibit a natural process that is integral to overall health, but antiperspirants contain aluminum, which is toxic; we thoughtlessly apply them to our underarms, where there are lymph nodes important for detoxification and the fighting of disease needlessly taxing their function. By contrast, encouraging sweating and unclogging pores through dry-brushing and body exfoliation aids detoxification, and when performed all over, also reduces cellulite.

The capillaries in the skin also transport debris such as bacteria, pollution, dead cells, and absorbed skin care ingredients to the heart to be cleared and filtered out. Keeping the walls of the blood vessels moist and supple through keeping the skin moisturized is important to this detoxification.

The skin is an organ of absorption; even a small percentage of our total oxygen intake is absorbed through our pores. This is why we must choose carefully what we put on our skin. What is applied topically travels into the bloodstream through a network of capillaries connecting to larger vessels that supply the internal organs. The skin actually absorbs materials faster than the digestive system. What we eat must be processed before it fully affects our health, but anything applied to the skin has direct access to our blood. Nicotine patches used to wean smokers from cigarettes are a good example of this.

The skin's absorptive ability can also be an avenue of healing and medication, as with prescription hormone creams used for hormonal supplementation. But topical therapy is not new to ayurveda. Topical treatment is a traditional part of practice that offers astonishing results. During a lecture at the Ayurvedic Academy at Bastyr University in Seattle, Washington, Dr. Subhash Ranade spoke of an experiment conducted in an underprivileged village in India. Starvation had damaged the digestive systems of many children, making it difficult for them to absorb nutrients from their food. These children were given a daily massage of milk infused with healing herbs, the absorption of which gradually restored the lining of their digestive tracts. The treatments these children absorbed through the skin made profound improvements in their weight and digestive systems.

When we understand how profound our ability to absorb through the skin is, we can begin to also comprehend the importance of choosing healthy skin and body care products. Many people may think of beauty care as only superficial and fun, yet its impact on the body as a holistic system is highly significant.

Skin Structure

To truly understand skin and how to keep it healthy, we must understand its makeup. Our skin is not just what we see; it is an entire factory, support system, and shield for a variety of vitally functioning cells. As shown in the diagram below, the skin is made up of three main layers: the epidermis, the dermis, and the hypodermis. The epidermis is the layer closest to the surface. It is the outer shell that we see, and it acts as both a barrier and a gateway. It is composed of five layers of dead skin cells made up of keratin (protein). Keratinization is the process by which cells travel up through these layers to become the surface. This process ends when the cells are eventually sloughed off. The life cycle of skin cells becomes slower over the years, producing the effects we call aging.

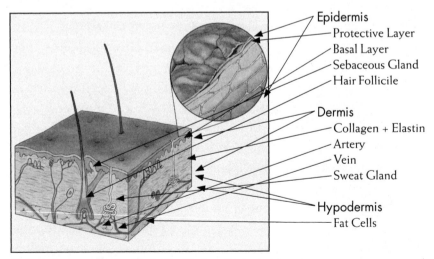

Epidermis
  Protective Layer
  Basal Layer
  Sebaceous Gland
  Hair Follicile

Dermis
  Collagen + Elastin
  Artery
  Vein
  Sweat Gland

Hypodermis
  Fat Cells

© iStockphoto.com/Dorling Kindersley (Dorling_Kindersley).

The layer beneath the epidermis is called the dermis. This is the main factory of the skin, containing its network of collagen and elastin fibers. The dermis's connective tissue provides elasticity and nutrition to the epidermis. The sweat and oil glands reside here, excreting through the epidermis. This layer also contains the nerve endings that provide our sense of touch and temperature. Its health dictates the quality of the epidermis.

Under the dermis layer is the hypodermis, also referred to as subcutaneous fatty tissue. This lowest layer of skin is the fatty cushion that insulates the body and protects the organs. Composed primarily of fat and some connective tissue, it also possesses many skin-nourishing blood vessels and nerve endings.

With age, the structure of the skin begins to change. As the quality and thickness of each layer alters, so do the skin's needs. At twenty-five, the skin is at its peak of health. The dermis layer is thick, producing lots of plump, moist cells to be transferred to the epidermis. Cell turnover takes approximately twenty-eight days. As we age, the epidermis thickens, giving way to fine lines and wrinkles as cell turnover slows down. By forty-five, the rate of this turnover decreases to approximately forty days. An accumulation of dead cells causes the skin to feel drier, and it is less able to absorb moisture.

At seventy-five, cell turnover drops further to ninety days, and the skin's metabolism and circulation also slow down. An even thicker epidermal layer causes wrinkles to deepen, with the top layer forming a crustlike appearance. This is why skin peeling and abrasion has become so popular. Exfoliation is one of the most result-oriented treatments for both rejuvenating skin and preventing signs of aging. The erosion of the thickened epidermis forces the dermis to increase cell production and sloughs away dead skin-cell buildup so the skin can absorb moisture more deeply.

Skin Classification

Now that we have an overview of the skin's nature and capabilities, we can discuss how to assess it and diagnose problems. To treat a problem, we need to classify and analyze it to find its root cause. Given that the body is so complex and that everyone is unique, different treatments are needed for each individual. This is the basis of ayurveda. When we can classify the skin and its imbalances from an ayurvedic perspective, we can identify its proper treatment and care. First, however, let us examine the different ways to diagnose skin from an esthetician's viewpoint.

THE CLASSIC SKIN TYPES

If you go to a department store cosmetics counter, the clerk will most likely base her suggestions on classic skin typing. This classification breaks each person into one of four categories: dry skin, oily skin, combination skin, and normal skin.

Dry skin lacks oil and has small pores and a fine texture. Because this skin type has little moisture, it may take on a leathery appearance during maturity. Dry skin is also said to be free from acne. In contrast, oily skin has (surprise!) an abundance of oil. Excess sebum is visible on the skin's surface, and this skin type also displays enlarged pores and a thick texture. It is not prone to fine lines, but eventual wrinkles appear as deep expression lines. Oily skin is said to be prone to acne.

Combination skin is a mixture of dry and oily skin types. Such complexions are oily in the T-zone area (the forehead, nose, and chin) and dry on the cheeks. Perfectly balanced skin is ironically referred to as normal, even though it's actually the least common skin type and denotes a flawless complexion.

Classic skin typing takes only the innate genetic characteristics of the skin into account; it does not consider environmental factors or past skin care efforts that may have caused sebaceous imbalance. It also looks only at the amount of oil in the skin, ignoring water content and other skin conditions. This classification alone is not effective in accurately diagnosing the skin.

SKIN TYPING BY CONDITION

While classic skin typing focuses on what skin qualities we've inherited, what beauty professionals call "skin conditions" refers to what we have acquired. This skin classification is based on environment and grooming history, and it also indicates that these conditions are reversible. Skin typing by condition most notably uses the terms "dehydrated skin," "sensitive skin," "unbalanced skin," and "problem skin."

Dehydrated skin is probably the most common skin condition and is due to a lack of water in the skin. This should not be confused with dry skin, which lacks oil. Dehydrated skin lacks water. This translates into many symptoms, such as a crepey or crinkled texture, lack of color, congested pores, and poor circulation. Dehydrated skin feels tight and sometimes rough. A lack of water weakens the skin and impairs its barrier function; it also contributes to many other skin ailments not regularly associated with skin dehydration. The best way to tell if your skin is dehydrated is to do a press test. Gently press the side of your cheek; if the surrounding area shows tiny lines, the skin is dehydrated.

Another common skin condition is sensitive skin. While this may be genetic, it is aggravated by the elements, diet, mind-set, and improper care. Inflammation caused by these factors results in redness, broken capillaries, and/or a chafed appearance. People with sensitive skin blush easily, and in more extreme cases, they may break out in rashes or hives when upset. Allergic skin is a type of sensitivity; while many may consider allergies unavoidable, ayurveda considers allergies to be an indication of internal toxicity. An overload of toxins makes our body delicate and weakens the defenses, leading to highly reactive skin all over the body.

Unbalanced skin indicates an imbalance in oil production. While this seems similar to the classic skin types, it is not genetic but is caused by overdrying, negligent skin care, or high stress levels (causing overactive adrenal glands). Unbalanced skin can take the form of oily skin that also peels; exhibits fine lines, dryness, or tightness combined with acne; or has whiteheads beneath the skin. (We will discuss this in more detail later in this chapter.) Unbalanced skin has usually been dehydrated for so long that the skin's attempt to rebalance causes dysfunction in the sebaceous glands.

Unbalanced skin conditions often lead to problem skin, which is "beautyspeak" for skin with pimples and blackheads. It is important to mention that this does not refer to one or two pimples but to a condition in which the skin constantly breaks out with acne and blemish clusters all over the face and sometimes the neck. Signs of problem skin include whiteheads, blackheads, inflamed pimples, and cystic acne. Causes vary from person to person and are discussed further in chapter 6.

Skin typing through skin condition only identifies what is out of balance with your complexion. From this point of view, you simply treat what needs to be "corrected" rather than deeply understanding the nature of the skin. For this reason, it is only one aspect of skin diagnosis, and other measures must be taken into consideration.

Female versus Male Skin

While many grooming practices are gender neutral, some differences cannot be ignored. Because of the nature of male and female skin, we must examine the influence of gender on skin structure and how it must be treated.

Men have thicker, tougher, and rougher skin than women do; even the most delicate male skin is much thicker and less sensitive than female skin. The male hormone testosterone increases collagen production, which is the main reason for the greater thickness. Estrogen decreases collagen synthesis but supports the presence of hyaluronic acid, which makes for a thinner, softer texture.

While male skin owes much to physiology, men also have a skin-thickening, antiaging practice ingrained in their grooming regimens from adolescence: shaving. This continual exfoliation acts the same way as microdermabrasion: it thickens the skin while it abrades it, causing regeneration. This is a major reason why men often have fewer fine lines and more vital skin. They also tend to have oilier skin. Because testosterone creates more active sebaceous glands, men are more prone to acne and breakouts. Women with hormonal imbalances also share these attributes.

For women, the same hormonal influences that cause menstruation can also cause preperiod breakouts, skin sensitivity, and water retention. According to ayurveda, this is because both water and heat in the body are increased before menstruation increasing inflammation and contributing to edema. Many women crave sweet, cooling foods at this time and have mood swings ranging from anger (heat aggravated) to feelings of lethargy (water aggravated).

Women are also more likely to have rosacea, although severe stages of the disease are usually only seen in men, due to neglect of care. Water retention during menstruation also contributes to sensitivity, because if the lymph is full, the capillaries are pushed toward the skin's surface. This pressure can create broken capillaries, further increasing the skin's delicacy. For all these reasons, women who want beautiful skin must pay attention to their menstrual cycles.

Master the Balancing Act of Oil and Water

When diagnosing the skin, it is beneficial to overlook the traditional categories of dry, oily, and combination, because many people with oil on the skin surface are actually dry-skinned and have self-induced the overproduction of oil. The opposite can also happen. Some people attempt to treat dryness by slathering on oil-rich products, when they really suffer from a lack of water.

The skin is constantly striving to be "normal." In the most basic terms, this means achieving a healthy balance of oil and water, which allows it to be a barrier, absorber, eliminator, and regenerator. When you know which (or both) you lack, it is easy to make skin care decisions to correct the imbalance. Just to clarify, we are going to be talking about skin care made with natural vegetable oils (organic, unprocessed ones are even better) and waters (preferably *hydrosols*: waters extracted from plants or flowers). Chemical-based systems only exacerbate the imbalance due to their stripping and congesting properties.

When I first started my practice, I quickly became aware of how important our water-to-oil ratio is. Maintaining skin health is basically balancing the water it contains and the protective oil that lubricates its surface. I found this method of looking at whether the skin was hydrated or dehydrated, and either oily or dry, far more useful than the traditional classifications I had learned in esthetics college.

Oily Dehydrated Skin

Oily dehydrated skin lacks water, making it feel tight yet greasy. Sometimes it flakes even though there is oil on the surface. It is prone to clogged pores, because the underlying lack of water causes the oil to dry and harden. A common misconception is that oily skin should never be moisturized; when in fact, it needs hydration to prevent it from overproducing sebum. Therefore, dehydration can be the real cause of acne.

During a facial, extraction (removal of blackheads and whiteheads) is difficult if the skin is dehydrated; often, a client needs to follow a hydrating regimen for at least two weeks before returning for a successful pore cleansing. This regimen must not strip the skin, so it should include a milk cleanser, because astringents can encourage oil production. If you prefer a gel cleanser, it must be gentle and not contain sodium laurel sulfate. Toners must be alcohol-free so as not to dry out the skin.

In addition to avoiding a dehydrating care regimen, those with an oily dehydrated skin also need to replenish with water. A serum is an excellent way to supplement hydration of the skin. This should be followed by a medium-weight moisturizer to seal in the water, slow down evaporation from the skin surface, and soften its texture. Because the skin has a good amount of oil in it to provide protection, it does not require anything too rich.

Oily Hydrated Skin

Oily hydrated skin is the traditional oily skin type. Do not fall into the misconception that this skin type needs to be dried out; it still needs protection and moisture to maintain its beauty. Oily hydrated skin ages well, and blackheads and whiteheads can be extracted easily. For this skin type, a light moisturizer is ideal. Sometimes a serum on its own can be sufficient in maintaining moisture during warm, humid months. One way to keep skin clear of impurities is to use a detoxifying clay mask once or twice a week. I like both wet and powder-based masks. While wet clay masks are easier to use, the powdered variety stays fresh longer.

Dry Dehydrated Skin

This skin type is very depleted and needs both oil and water; hydration is quickly lost through both evaporation and loss of collagen. Any blackheads or whiteheads are tiny and difficult to extract, and this type of skin tends to show signs of aging earlier than other types. Those with dry dehydrated skin should use a milk cleanser and start using an antiaging serum at a young age. Serums that contain collagen, hyaluronic acid, or other plumping ingredients are especially beneficial and should be followed by a rich, nourishing cream. The cream protects the skin, replaces oil content, and closes off the skin to retain the water from the serum.

Dry Hydrated Skin

Dry hydrated skin is genetically oil-poor but still full of water. This usually occurs in younger people with a traditional dry skin type. Pores are small, and the skin looks thin but is actually healthy, plump, and hydrated. Because its surface is dry, it needs oil. Sometimes a face oil or rich cream on its own can be enough. Usually this condition is only temporary, because as the skin ages, it naturally loses collagen and holds less water, making it dry and dehydrated.

Combination Hydrated Skin

This skin type is generally healthy and similar to the oily hydrated type. While combination hydrated skin will most likely have excess oil in the T-zone, there is nothing wrong with extra sebaceous secretions in this area—the hydration usually prevents the skin from becoming congested.

If the skin does break out or the pores become clogged, regular facials can clear the pores in the T-zone without overpeeling or drying the entire face. Another way to help keep this mixed skin type in balance is by using an organic lavender hydrosol (lavender water) as a toner. This hydrates the skin by replenishing water, while the lavender purifies, balances oil, and has a slight antiseptic quality. A medium-weight cream should be used following the toner.

COMBINATION DEHYDRATED SKIN

The lack of water in combination dehydrated skin makes it prone to several problems. This type of skin is oily in the T-zone but dry on the cheeks. Pores are easily blocked due to the lack of water. Mixing and/or layering serums and creams as described for dry, dehydrated skin is important here. We can mix these two moisturizing steps or apply each in the specific areas needed.

Those with combination dehydrated skin may find that when the moisture level of the skin is increased, the contrast in oiliness between the T-zone and the rest of the face is reduced.

NORMAL SKIN

Perfectly normal skin simply needs gentle maintenance to prevent future imbalances, but using a natural skin care regimen is important to prevent causing other skin conditions. Gentle, neutral cleansers and toners (not treatment based) are therapeutic enough to keep this skin type healthy. Never use bar soap, as it encourages dehydration. This is an across-the-board rule for all skin types, but it is easily ignored when you have beautiful, normal skin. A simple, medium-weight, natural moisturizer is you need for this perfectly balanced complexion. In dry, cold climates, a facial oil can also be used.

Ayurveda and Skin Type

Understanding skin type according to dosha is not limited to the skin's oil content, the damage it has acquired, or its hydration levels. Rather when identifying complexions ayurvedically, we look at genetic predispositions, the root or unique cause of the skin's reactions, and doshic tendencies. While the concept of balancing the skin's oil and water was enlightening to me as an esthetician, incorporating ayurveda into skin diagnosis looked at my client's predispositions to different imbalances and allowed me to prevent them.

This section describes the ayurvedic skin types and their qualities and conditions. Here we will learn how to identify our own doshic skin type, which will help us understand how to rebalance it, preventing skin ailments. It will also tell us about our overall body, mind, and spirit.

KAPHA SKIN

Kapha skin is easily the most beautiful skin type when it is in balance. It is thick, oily, and full of moisture, and it has a beautiful clarity of color. Again, the presence of earth and water are translated into the quality of the skin tissue, and the good amount of fatty tissue underlying it makes it firmer, moister, and more resilient to the signs of aging than the other two doshic skin types.

Kapha types usually have large pores brimming with oil, but remember that oiliness is not bad for the skin. It is only when oil is combined with a lack of water that skin issues occur. When kapha skin becomes dehydrated, it becomes the most problematic skin type. Oil dries on the surface, forming deposits of hardened sebum in the pores. This gives way to comedones (blackheads), enlarged pores, and blemishes. This skin type also has a tendency toward pimples with kapha qualities—they are large, full of fluid, and often leave deep scars that alter the skin's structure. Kapha skin can scar so severely that its surface is altered by "ice pick scars," indentations that are very difficult to treat.

Dehydration also causes an excess of oil. So when kapha skin becomes dehydrated, the sebaceous glands produce more oil to compensate for the lack of moisture. Not only does it create more oil, but the oil itself becomes heavier and thicker.

Kapha complexions tend to accumulate lymphatic fluid which creates puffiness. Excess kapha can inhibit circulation and promote lymphatic congestion, causing a moonfaced look. This lack of drainage and propensity toward stagnation also can result in dull-looking skin.

Another symptom of too much kapha is thick skin. Regardless of your prakruti, if there is an overabundance of earth and water in your vikruti, the skin on your cheeks and chin can become thick in appearance. This is usually coupled with dehydration and enlarged pores, creating an "orange peel effect" (thickened texture with visible pores) on the skin's surface.

Because kaphas tend to be lackadaisical about their grooming habits, it is important to try to be strict about regular care. Sometimes imbalance can come from sheer lack of attention or being inconsistent with cleansing, toning, and moisturizing. This can contribute to the transition from innately beautiful skin to skin that is overly oily with clogged pores.

To keep kapha skin beautiful and balanced, you must concentrate on keeping the skin hydrated and the circulation moving. Using skin care products with purifying ingredients such as sage, eucalyptus, and rosemary helps keep kapha skin clear and stimulated. Vitamin C, honey, and citrus ingredients are other great additives for kapha as they are invigorating and prevent aging by increasing hydration and promoting collagen production.

Pitta Skin

Pitta skin is sensitive and easily inflamed. It is prone to allergic reactions, rashes, eczema, acne, and rosacea. When the capillaries are overactive and dilated, this indicates an excess of pitta in the body and skin; it is also why those with high pitta have a tendency toward broken capillaries and blood vessels, especially in the cheeks and nose.

Pitta skin is a combination type when it comes to oil production (only in the T-zone), with a medium-thick texture and medium-size pores. One sign of excess heat is enlarged pores in the midface that are so dehydrated that the blockages are difficult to extract. Using a cooling, hydrating moisturizer containing an anti-inflammatory ingredient such as aloe vera or rosewater helps soften these pores and minimize their appearance. According to ayurveda, those with too much internal inflammation are prone to dehydration because internal heat burns up the body's water supply. This further contributes to a pitta's skin sensitivity and makes blemishes worse.

Pitta skin also scars easily and tends toward changes in pigmentation. Unlike kapha skin, this is in the form of marks and discoloration rather than detexturization. Hyperpigmentation is created by inflammation that disrupts the production of melanin (the pigment that gives skin its color). Because pitta governs transformation and assimilation, the transfer of melanin from melanocytes at the bottom layer of the epidermis to keratinocytes in the middle and top layers is also a pitta activity. Excess pitta disrupts the process of skin color distribution, causing dark spots, freckles, and pigmented lesions.

Those with pitta skin must maintain balance by using soothing skin care products that contain chamomile, calendula, and sandalwood. These are wonderfully calming, anti-inflammatory ingredients.

Most oils and fats induce heat and should be avoided when pitta is overabundant, but coconut oil is actually cooling. Jojoba is another substance that can be used, because although it is often mistaken for an oil, pure jojoba actually contains no fat and therefore does not increase fire. Rosehip oil can also be used for some pitta skin types. It is one of the only natural ingredients that successfully fades pigmented spots and scars and treats sun damage. But this oil is slightly stimulating and should be used as a spot treatment for only a short time to strengthen and diminish hyperpigmentation and scarring. It should not be used on acne-prone complexions.

Ghee is another moisturizing ingredient that can bring down both internal and topical heat. Ghee is a clarified butter and a traditional ayurvedic remedy for rashes and other skin reactions.

Vata Skin

Vata skin has small, tight pores; a thin texture; and a lack of oil. Because this skin type does not have much fat behind its tissue, it is easily depleted and can begin to sag early. When those with vata skin are young, they do not usually have a problem with blemishes or oiliness. Instead, the skin can appear so clear and delicate that the veins and capillaries show through it faintly. (This does not refer to red, broken blood vessels but to the bluish blood pathways under the skin.)

Unfortunately, vatas are prone to other premature signs of aging besides sagging. As you age, the skin thins, facial fat decreases, and collagen production slows down. Because this skin type is already lacking in tissue and oil, it has less reserves against the aging process than those associated with the other two doshas. Even if you do not have a vata prikruti, if you accumulate too much stress and vata energy, your skin will show vata characteristics—a loss of firmness and plumpness, a decrease in oil content, and internal and external dehydration. For this reason, those with high vata need to work on becoming more grounded and less cerebral, nurturing the connection between mind and body.

When it comes to a skin care regimen, vata skin must be nourished, nourished, nourished! It is important to use products with warming and rejuvenating ingredients like ginseng, frankincense, and ylang-ylang.

Geranium oil is also good for vata as it has fabulous antiaging properties and helps relieve anxiety.

Rich oils are vata's best friend and using liberal amounts of avocado, sesame, borage, and evening primrose oils helps fight dryness and replenishes this skin type. Rosehip oil is excellent for vata skin, as it is slightly stimulating and possesses high amounts of vitamin C, making it a great antioxidant moisturizer. Vatas should apply these oils on both the body and the face to nourish the skin as an organ and to help support, warm, and ground the body as a whole. Vatas need more than just moisturizing with oils; this skin type is so delicate that it also must address dehydration. As with the dry dehydrated skin type described earlier in this chapter, the most effective way to support vata skin is by layering fatty oils over a water-packed serum. A serum with collagen helps bolster depleted skin, and products containing hyaluronic acid can help hydrate the skin.

Identifying your ayurvedic skin type helps you understand categories of characteristics instead of concentrating only on oil content, present appearance, or a specific ailment. When you see your skin from this angle, you are more likely to treat your skin and body with appropriate care products and are better able to maintain internal balance for more beautiful skin.

This holistic approach also illustrates why a skin care regimen needs to be individually tailored according to both topical condition and your ayurvedic constitution. In the next section of this book, we'll examine what makes up a truly effective skin care routine, the role of facial treatments, advances in natural cosmetic options, and skin care guidance for each of the three doshas.

Part Two

SKIN CARE MADE PURE AND SIMPLE

Four

Skin Care 101

Now that we have talked about how to diagnose your skin and treat problems, we need to examine the way you care for your skin on a daily basis. Often, we do not know what skin care items to use and how many steps our beauty regime should include. This next section aims to distill this information and provide simple guidelines and reasoning to clarify what goes into an effective beauty routine.

The Basic Regimen

A basic skin care regimen includes cleansing, toning, and moisturizing. This keeps the skin clear of dirt, debris, and toxins as well as supports and protects it. Beyond this, the eye area, lips, and chest require special care, and there are extra rituals, such as exfoliation, masks, and professional facials, that give our skin added support when it has become out of balance. But first, let us determine what to look for in everyday skin care.

CLEANSING

Cleansing the skin, day and night, to remove buildup and grime is the first step of a proper skin care routine. We must start with a clean surface before applying a barrier or layers of moisture.

During sleep, the skin excretes toxins, so cleansing in the morning helps get rid of these impurities. During the day, it is exposed to so much pollution that evening cleansing is necessary to wash away the dirt that congests the pores. Clients have asked me if it is necessary to cleanse both day and night, and while I think doing so is important, if I had to choose one over the other, the evening facial cleanse is more essential. This is because pollution residue on the skin actually creates free radicals, which in turn causes signs of aging and damage.

I have also been asked if rinsing with water is sufficient, but unfortunately, water alone does not have the fatty material needed to break down oil-soluble impurities. Of course, you do not want to overwash, so a gentle cleanser that does not contain sodium laurel sulfate (SLS, which strips the acid mantle) is important whatever your skin type.

Selecting the right cleanser is important as it is the initial step of your facial regime. You need to make sure you are cleansing according to your skin type to enable all other products to work properly and maintain balance.

Vata types should use a rich, milky cleanser that will help maintain the skin's moisture. Because this skin type is prone to premature aging and skin depletion, it is important not to use anything too astringent. Cleansing products that contain ingredients that increase circulation are also beneficial. When you increase circulation, you increase collagen production, and because vata skin has a naturally thin texture, supporting collagen in the skin is imperative.

Pitta skin also needs a milk cleanser, but make sure the product is not so rich that it still has good viscosity. Cleansers for pitta skin types should be light and lotionlike, because heavy oils can stimulate heat. Pitta skin has a lot of heat, so natural cleansers for sensitive skin are ideal. These products contain calming, soothing ingredients like rose essential oil, rose water, chamomile, and aloe vera.

Kaphas can use a gel cleanser that lathers slightly, but avoid any product that foams heavily as it most likely contains SLS. This skin type is thick and oily with easily clogged pores, so a cleanser that provides deep cleansing is best. Kaphas whose complexion is especially dull or broken out and who are not sensitive can also try a cleanser that contains peeling ingredients. Choose one geared toward gentle purifying, with ingredients such as sage, lavender, and peppermint that will disinfect the skin and help prevent kapha accumulation.

Toning

A toner tightens the pores, keeping out pollution, bacteria, and dirt. In the past, toners were primarily used to clean off residue from petroleum-based cleansers. Since this is not necessary with petroleum-free products, today's toners are more beneficial for hydration, balancing the skin's pH, and contracting pores. A good hydrating toner also helps other products penetrate the skin. According to ayurveda, oils and other moisturizing ingredients penetrate more deeply into moist skin. You may think absorption can be promoted by simply applying moisturizer to a wet face, but water does not provide the pH balance that a toner made expressly for this purpose does. Not only does a good natural toner promote healthy skin through pH balance (striving for pH 5.0–5.6, which also prevents acne as germs do not grow in acidic environments), but the slight oiliness from its plant ingredients aids penetration better than simple H_2O.

Like any other product, most toners have specific uses. For example, hydrosols (waters extracted from plants and flowers) of chamomile or rose are great for calming inflammation (ideal for pitta skin), whereas a yarrow hydrosol or toner with collagen have antiaging properties (ideal for vatas). If you need to prevent breakouts or bacterial infection (kapha skin), your toner must not contain drying ingredients like alcohol;

organic witch hazel, peppermint, and sage hydrosols are great for disinfecting without stripping, irritating, or extracting moisture. Witch hazel is especially good because it also reduces inflammation.

Using a cotton pad to apply toner unfortunately wastes both the cotton and the toner. I recommend misting; this method is simple and hygienic and also saves product. Many toners today come in packaging with a misting nozzle, but if yours doesn't, you can simply transfer the product to a spray bottle.

Moisturizing

Moisturizers serve two purposes: hydration and protection. Since the skin naturally contains oil and water, proper moisturizing comes from products that contain both ingredients. Beyond providing hydration and protection, moisturizers usually have secondary properties and contain other ingredients that stimulate, add minerals, or disinfect the skin.

Moisturizing often involves more than one product. For dehydrated skin types, using a serum under a rich cream enhances the overall effect. Since oil does not hydrate, and water and serums give little protection, a serum and a cream provide a wonderful combination. Serums also contribute to the skin's barrier function, because plump skin cells help guard against water loss and make skin structure more dense. Layering products is especially good for those who travel often or live in environments with fluctuating weather. This two-step moisturizing process enables you to tailor each day's regimen to your skin's needs based on internal and external conditions. If the climate is humid or your skin is well hydrated, you can forgo the serum; when you are sensitive or inflamed, you can omit the oil/cream or switch to a lotion.

Weather greatly influences the doshas, so it also affects the complexion. Skin behaves differently according to its surroundings and the seasons. While many people may make adjustments intuitively, it is important to remember that dry, cold conditions call for heavier, more nourishing skin care and warm, wet conditions require lighter products. Once you understand this, you can begin to monitor how your skin interacts with its environment and change your regimen from day to day, just as you change your clothing, to suit the weather. A heavy moisturizing cream, like a heavy winter coat, protects skin from the elements, whereas a light lotion, like a light spring jacket, provides some resistance to the elements but allows skin to breathe more easily on warm days.

There is also the issue of choosing a day and a night cream. Although I personally use the same moisturizers for both, many of my clients have benefitted from using separate products. During the day, when you are exposed to the elements and often apply makeup or sunblock, you may wish to choose a lighter cream. Many of my clients are concerned about their skin looking shiny or oily, but they have skin types that need a rich cream or face oil. They compromise by using a light moisturizer during the day and a heavier one at night.

Traditionally, night creams are heavier in texture than day creams, because the skin can absorb and digest larger molecules at night. While feeding the skin at night can be effective, many skin care companies no longer advocate this. They believe that the skin detoxifies and purges toxins during sleep as the body regenerates and suggest omitting a nighttime moisturizer altogether. While the elimination of nightly moisturizing may leave the skin feeling dry for the first two weeks, the skin will gradually adjust. Again, you can compromise by using a light moisturizer, serum, or concentrated liquid ampoule to give your skin some moisture while allowing the process of detoxification to occur.

Ultimately, the use of night creams depends on the individual. If the skin is severely depleted, nighttime nourishment is excellent, especially for those (like acne sufferers) who dislike the feeling of oiliness or heaviness during the day. Bedtime moisturizing is also advisable when a dry climate is involved. I'm from Canada, and the harsh winters suck moisture from the skin. The cold conditions force people to reside in dry, heated environments that also take their toll on the complexion and require as much replenishment as possible. But for those who live in more humid climates, opting for a light night product is helpful to keep the skin healthy and the pores open.

The moisturizing step is probably the most important, since the moisturizer stays on the skin all day and helps support its equilibrium. Selecting a moisturizer can be difficult because there are so many factors involved—even the number of steps in the process can depend on the state of the skin.

Looking at the skin's doshic imbalance is the best way to choose a moisturizing routine. Those with a lot of vata in their skin experience a lack of both water and oil, so they need to use a water-rich serum as well as a rich cream to seal the water in. Sometimes, I even recommend a face oil on top of these two layers if an individual has extremely depleted skin. All moisturizing products should contain antiaging ingredients like collagen or other circulation-stimulating ingredients such as ginseng or ginger root. The best oils to look for in a rich cream or facial oil product are sesame, avocado, borage, and evening primrose. Traditionally, ayurveda uses sesame oil for vata afflictions, but avocado is wonderfully rich and nourishing, borage is restorative and helps repair skin damage, and evening primrose is excellent for antiaging and supporting women going through menopause (vata transition).

Pitta skin also needs a serum and a moisturizer. Because pitta is the fire dosha, a water-based serum helps decrease fire and soothes the skin. If your face is broken out with a rash or an allergic reaction, you should avoid products with too much oil and opt instead to apply a serum several times a day. You should also switch to a light lotion, which contains less oil than a cream. When pitta is under control, a moisturizer that contains coconut oil and/or jojoba is good for maintaining the balance and managing heat.

Kapha skin only needs the added step of a serum if it is dehydrated. When this happens, the skin is actually influenced by a vata imbalance. Otherwise, a light to medium-weight lotion is the best option. Look for ingredients that promote circulation, as this helps prevent lymphatic congestion in the skin. If kapha skin feels overly oily, this can also be an indication of too much vata that induces the body to produce more oil. Again, sesame oil is an excellent lotion ingredient, since it is therapeutic to both vata and kapha, but hazelnut oil is another great option, because it helps rebalance overactive sebaceous glands.

Caring for the Eyes, Lips, and Neck/Upper Chest

The skin of the eyes, lips, and neck/chest is delicate and needs special care. It is often thinner and more easily injured, and these areas are the first to show signs of aging. These fragile parts of the body also divulge many facets of our internal health and can reveal early imbalances and indications of disease.

EYES: THE WINDOWS TO THE SOUL

Your eyes are one of the first things others notice about you, and while the saying goes that they are windows to the soul, they are also windows to your health. You can learn a lot about your health through iridology (reading the iris to diagnose health) and ayurveda. When your eyes are bright and alert, they reflect an astuteness and a clarity of mind; when they are cloudy or tired, they display imbalance. Bloodshot or yellowed eyes indicate pitta *ama* (toxicity) in the body, whereas brown spots can indicate parasites. The skin around the eyes also tells a story. As discussed in the face mapping section of chapter 2, the area beneath the eyes is related to the kidneys, and undereye bags or darkness can be attributed to weakness in these organs.

Coincidentally, the eyes are also one of the first areas to show signs of aging. Because we often overwork them, they are prone to exhaustion. There are many outrageously expensive eye creams and treatments on the market, demonstrating just how much we treasure beautiful eyes.

Sensitive Eyes: Many of us have sensitive eyes due to genetics, eyestrain, or poor daily care. Since the eyes are the domain of pitta, which governs heat, redness, irritation, and inflammation, sensitive eyes—with their dryness and burning sensations—are related to excess pitta. People who work with and care for many patients throughout the day, such as massage therapists, health practitioners, and estheticians, have a higher tendency for accumulating pitta in the eyes, because they pick up heat from the many individuals they touch and interact with. One ayurvedic remedy for eyes that become easily inflamed is castor oil drops, which help dissipate and purge excess heat. Put one to two drops of pure castor oil in each eye every night for calm, less sensitive eyes.

From a more conventional standpoint, sensitive eyes can be treated with a cooling, hydrating eye cream or gel. A water-rich product is key; oil-rich eye products are more warming and should only be used by those who are less prone to eye inflammation. Cool compresses soaked with rosewater or chamomile water also reduce heat in the eyes.

Many people with sensitive eyes may be allergic to the ingredients or preservatives in eye products, but sometimes stinging can be mistaken for a reaction when it is just an initial response to the product's cooling properties. If stinging dissipates quickly, the eyes are simply adjusting to the anti-inflammatory action.

When using eye makeup, less is usually more if you have sensitive eyes. Mineral eye shadows and liners made of pure ingredients are the products to choose, because they do not contain irritating dyes. Organic kajal eyeliners are best for allergy-prone eyes. Traditional ayurvedic kajals are cream liners (usually black in color) made from the carbon of burnt ghee; they are completely natural, and ghee is a powerful anti-inflammatory.

Dark Circles: There are many causes for "raccoon eyes," but most people assume it is a genetic trait because it's something they've had for as long as they can remember. Undereye circles may be inherited, but the genetics that cause them may affect the kidneys more than the eyes.

In ayurvedic diagnosis, the lower lid is an adrenal area, and lower than this—where the eye socket begins—is a kidney area (feel the bone under your eye). As you get older, the skin around your eyes gets more saggy and baggy, with dark circles becoming more pronounced. This is because the kidneys are vata organs, and the vata dosha becomes much stronger in maturity and old age. Those with high vata often have undereye discoloration even from a young age.

Another cause of dark circles is deoxygenated blood. Blood without oxygen is dark, which causes bluishness under the eyes. Using products with antioxidants and eye creams that promote circulation can be very effective to counteract this. Arnica, along with other stimulating plants, is excellent. Arnica also helps drain lymphatic fluid and moves stagnant blood that causes undereye circles.

Puffy Eyes: Puffiness is a kapha trait. Any glandular or sinus congestion or other type of fluid retention is governed by the water element. Puffiness in the face is a combination of excess water in the body combined with the presence of heat; heat rises, bringing water retention into the upper body. If heat is not strong, the water retention is found only in the lower body, most notably in the legs and ankles. So puffy eyes are an indication of excess kapha and pitta elements/toxins.

Lack of sleep also makes the eyes puffy, because the lower eyelid corresponds to the adrenal glands and kidneys. Though affected by the adrenals, the kidneys are also important for filtering and absorbing water into the body. Inadequate sleep leads to a vata-induced kapha-pitta imbalance.

Puffy eyes can also be attributed to constipation. When the body is not emptied of waste, it holds turbid water and increases kapha energy. Because the kapha dosha is heavy and sluggish, this contributes further to the lack of movement in the bowels. Ensuring proper and full elimination helps decrease facial edema and water retention.

Kapha is strongest in the morning, and this is usually when your face looks most bloated and puffy. As the day wears on, you become more active and stimulated, so the puffiness drains away. To accelerate this, give yourself a pressure-point massage while washing your face in the morning. Press gently around the bones of the eye socket in a circular pattern, then gently press and release the other swollen sinus areas. Engaging in this lymph-drainage massage every morning helps my own kapha puffiness subside. Exercising early in the day also moves lymph and stimulates drainage.

Cholesterol/Fat Deposits: Sometimes we acquire little whiteheads near the eye area. These bumps—referred to as cholesterol or fat deposits—sit on the skin and are so difficult to extract that they can often only be removed when punctured with a needle. Only trained professionals should do this since the delicacy of the eye area makes it easy to bruise the skin or break capillaries. Fat deposits can be caused by a number of things, but most often they are the result of using pore-clogging skin care products. Because the pores in this area of the face are smaller, it is important to use a natural eye cream that will not block them. As we've discussed in other chapters, when buildup accumulates in dehydrated skin, it dries and hardens in the pores.

Cholesterol/fat deposits can also be due to toxins or excess fat in the internal organs. This results from a high-fat diet or the inability of the body to flush cholesterol. Most often it is a combination of clogged pores and internal problems that cause these deposits. Fat deposits may disappear when you switch to a more natural, non-clogging eye cream or gel, but I advise pairing this with a kidney cleanse or some other type of detox treatment.

LIPS: PRETTY POUTS

Since the lips contain more delicate tissue than the rest of the face, they are often the first to show an allergic reaction. Because they relate to the digestive system, swelling, itchiness, and irritation can indicate an internal problem. Swollen lips are a sign of extreme dehydration in the intestines and/or stomach and indicate the body's attempt to retain water.

While most people see dry or flaky lips as a normal result of the winter season, they indicate a need for internal and external hydration. You can hydrate the gastrointestinal tract by eating a water-rich, easy-to-digest diet. For further diagnosis and recommendations, you may benefit from consulting a health practitioner.

Topical protection for dry lips is essential. Using mass-market lip balms with petrolatum is often counterproductive, because they congest the lips' pores instead of penetrating the tissue. This is why many people become addicted to Chapstick; we love the sensation of moisture, but when that wears off, we are left with extreme dryness that needs another application. Balms made of vegetable butters, waxes, and oils are much more nourishing and still offer protection.

The Neck and Upper Chest

We often neglect the neck and upper chest, where the delicate, thinner skin is more prone to sagging, sun damage, and wrinkling. While it is not necessary to buy products specifically for the neck, I do recommend caring for it with serums and creams as religiously as you do your face. I use my face care regime on my chest. SPF protection with a mineral-based sunblock is especially important and should be applied daily, since this area is so vulnerable to sun exposure.

As we age, the skin on the front of the neck may begin to sag. This is mostly due to loss of tightness and strength in the neck muscles. Facial exercises can help sustain firmness here. Contracting and releasing an overexaggerated smile, as well as pushing the chin and head forward and back (I call this the "turkey move"), strengthen the muscles under the jawline and down the neck.

Premature skin sagging or formation of a double chin can also be due to an enlarged thyroid caused by mild hypothyroidism. While the aforementioned exercises help stimulate and bring circulation to the thyroid gland, seeking guidance on this issue from an ayurvedic physician can both alleviate this beauty concern and, through a holistic approach, improve the overall health of the endocrine system.

Extended Rituals

Beyond regular cleansing, toning, and moisturizing—along with care of the eye, lip, and chest areas—additional extended rituals can help keep the skin in balance. Unlike the necessity of a daily routine, extended rituals can be done as infrequently as once a week and act as supplementary support for the skin. The following at-home treatments are not too strenuous and can serve as little therapies that encourage you to take time out during the week for self-care and rejuvenation.

EXFOLIATION

Regular exfoliation keeps skin vibrant and young by eliminating dry, dead skin cells and promotes circulation. When you experience dull, devitalized skin, the fastest way to reenergize the look of your complexion is through exfoliation, which also helps prevent clogged pores and dehydration. Because pore congestion prevents the absorption of moisturizing products, a regular scrub or peel helps clear away this obstruction. Exfoliating products come in many different forms, and the frequency and depth of the treatment used depends on your skin type.

Vatas can exfoliate frequently with a gentle peeling product. If your skin is damaged with age spots and a leathery texture, you can even exfoliate every day. Of course, the peeling agent must be gentle. When using a nonabrasive peel such as a fruit acid, the percentage of acid should be low, and the product should also contain other restorative ingredients and antioxidants. If you use an abrasive exfoliant, it should be very finely ground. I often recommend a scrub that also contains lemon essential oil. Lemon is a natural exfoliant and bleaching agent, and when used in small amounts, it helps rejuvenate and brighten vata skin and increase circulation.

Pitta skin types cannot exfoliate as often, up to three times a week at most, and the product used should be extremely gentle. The one I recommend most often is a scrub made up of jojoba pearls (wax beads). This skin type can also use something as simple and easy to find as baking soda (sodium bicarbonate), which is alkaline. It makes the skin less acidic and also dissolves in water, making it a gentle exfoliant when applied to wet skin.

But pitta skin can also be prone to acne, and if your skin has pimples and bacteria on the surface, a nonabrasive exfoliant is much better than a granular scrub, which can break open pustules and infect the skin further. Again, a product containing a fruit acid– or sugar cane–derived glycolic acid is effective, but its use should be guided by a professional esthetician. Depending on how sensitive you skin is, you may only be able to use an exfoliant once a week.

Kapha skin is the thickest and most hardy of all three dosha types. It should be exfoliated often and deeply to reap the benefits of its natural beauty. Either nonabrasive peels or scrubs work well. Because of kapha skin's propensity toward dampness, I often recommend a dry exfoliant powder made of chickpea flour or ground olive shells. This provides an in-depth scrub, helps absorb excess oil, and promotes circulation by giving the exfoliant an added friction.

Masks

Although there are many different kinds of masks on the market, they can usually be broken down into three types: detoxifying/drying masks, nourishing/hydrating masks, and exfoliating masks. Recently, stimulating masks have become more common for promoting circulation, but they are not used regularly yet.

Masks are great tools for deep skin treatments. If you are going through unusual skin imbalances, a good therapeutic mask can help put your complexion back on track. I always recommend traveling with a powerful hydrating mask. Because air travel can dry the skin, using a replenishing mask as soon as you arrive at your destination helps prevent a breakout of eczema or prolonged dehydration.

I recommend that acne-prone clients always keep a clay mask in their medicine cabinet. Because acne is one of those skin conditions that fluctuates in severity, a clay mask helps dry and draw out impurities when a bad breakout occurs. It can also be used only as an overnight spot treatment on the blemishes alone. But since a clay mask can dry out the skin, I also suggest mixing it with a nourishing cream mask or hydrating gel mask. This is what we do at Pure + simple during facial treatments. This way we can tailor a mask to clients' skin conditions, depending on whether they have a combination of blemishes and sensitivity or blemishes and dehydration.

Kapha skin leans toward detoxifying/drying masks (which are usually clay masks), while pitta and vata skin use nourishing/hydrating masks (in either cream or gel form). Both vata and kapha skin can benefit from stimulating masks (the stimulation usually being provided by a spice ingredient such as wasabi or chili pepper), and all three skin types can use an exfoliating mask. Exfoliating masks are excellent if you don't have much time, because they nourish as well as peel. While there are many results-oriented, acid peeling masks, I especially like scrub masks. Because you apply the mask and let the ingredients sit and absorb, it often makes for deeper exfoliation. The skin also becomes less irritated when the mask is scrubbed off, because the skin is nicely hydrated, which decreases heat and sensitivity.

FACIALS

I love facials. With air travel being the fastest-growing source of greenhouse emissions and cruise ships producing an average of one hundred thousand liters of sewage per day, an all-natural spa day provides a local, eco-friendly "minivacation." The facials you can enjoy on one of these breaks tone the skin through stimulation and purification and are part of any proactive skin care routine.

A good facial should detoxify the skin and pores, move the blood, stimulate the lymphatic system and facial muscles, and nourish and treat the skin. Habitual facials are integral to keeping the skin in balance and clearing it of impurities, and those who need only simple maintenance should ideally have a facial every four to six weeks. Acne-prone skin may need a treatment every two to three weeks for more vigorous pore cleansing. Those who are actively combating signs of aging may want weekly treatments geared toward individual goals.

A classic European facial includes cleansing, exfoliation, steaming, extraction, facial massage, a mask, toning, and moisturizing. While some treatments may also incorporate bodywork or different kinds of exfoliation, a good, complete, basic facial should include all these steps.

That said, your skin may need a more specific approach based on your skin care needs and desires. I encourage you to discuss your beauty goals with your esthetician before your facial so he or she can choose the best products and techniques for you. The esthetician may also suggest other treatments, such as light-emitting diode therapy, facial acupuncture, or a specialized mask.

Every facial starts with cleansing the skin. This opens the ritual, clearing away makeup, pollution, excess sebum, and skin care product residue in order to prevent contamination. Cleansing during a facial should be gentle, nonstripping, and nondisruptive to the skin's acid mantle.

This is followed by exfoliation, which is actually an extension of the cleansing process aimed at clearing away dead cells and congestion. While some treatments may use a granular peel, others use alpha hydroxy acid (AHA), gommage, or sea-salt microdermabrasion. This polishes the skin, helping pore extraction by unclogging and moisturizing. At Pure + simple, we exfoliate under steam, because moist skin is less easily irritated. After sloughing away the dead skin cells and exposing new ones, we rehydrate and replenish the skin with a serum and oil. In rare cases, we do not exfoliate clients with highly sensitive skin; we simply apply collagen and oil under steam to minimize redness during extractions and to prepare the skin for the next process.

Steaming can be done after or during exfoliation. This is beneficial for opening and softening the pores because it hydrates the skin. Some people with sensitive skin may prefer to skip the steam, but instead of ignoring the entire step, I suggest applying rosewater pads to sensitive areas as a barrier. If you don't have these, try simply moving the steam further away so it emits less heat and force. I recommend always steaming during a facial, because the hydration and pore opening lessen the inflammation from extractions.

Every good facial should involve thorough extractions. This purging of toxins is vital to prevent stagnation and further enlargement of the pores. Keep in mind that a "good" extraction does not equate to an "aggressive" extraction; it purifies the skin carefully and meticulously. An experienced esthetician knows where to press on the skin and how much pressure is enough for each condition so there is never scarring or bruising. I usually advise clients not to try to do extractions themselves, because they are often unaware of how to do it properly; they may be too harsh and so determined to remove a blackhead or whitehead that they end up causing trauma to the skin. Plus, professional estheticians have better visibility because they use a magnifying lamp.

After extractions, the skin should be replenished and comforted with a gentle face massage. Not only is this wonderfully relaxing, but it also stimulates the circulation and the facial muscles while draining the lymph system and tissues of excess fluid. Different techniques have specific effects on the skin. Vigorous, upward movements are excellent for stimulating collagen and elastin production; slow, gentle, downward strokes are good for lymphatic drainage. In a technique called tapotement, oil is applied to the skin and then drummed in lightly with the fingertips. Of course, any massage should be done with a natural face oil that corresponds to your skin type.

The massage is followed by a mask that is individualized to each person's needs. As mentioned earlier, different types of masks can be mixed together to treat more than one skin condition. For example, an aloe vera–based, soothing gel mask combined with a detoxifying French clay mask can be used for congested, sensitive skin. While the mask dries, you can relax, exhale, and enjoy the stress-relieving benefits of your minivacation.

The facial treatment ends with toning and moisturizing, because the skin must always be protected before it is exposed to the environment. This is especially true in urban settings. As with each of the preceding steps, toning and moisturizing should address individual needs. If a treatment is performed during the day, the esthetician must also apply sunblock or mineral makeup for protection.

BODYCARE

Facials do not necessarily involve only the skin on the face. A truly holistic facial experience encompasses some body massage and helps restore the mind, body, and spirit. The emotional and spiritual rejuvenation that a treatment like this offers also translates into physical results. When the mind is at peace, the body becomes attuned to this state and can be open to true healing.

A facial that also treats the body provides full-body stimulation, promotes circulation and lymphatic drainage, moisturizes, and treats all skin as a single organ. The choice of body oils should match each person's doshic constitution. While vatas benefit from the warmth and richness of sesame oil, pittas can be calmed and soothed by anti-inflammatory oils such as coconut. Because kaphas are prone to chills and poor circulation, stimulating sesame oil is good, but mustard seed oil is best for a powerful boost of heat and movement in the fat cells.

If you can't afford or take time for a professional facial service or body massage, you must still pamper yourself with at-home body care.

When you massage oil into your body and scalp, you also boost moisture in your facial skin.

The skin is the largest organ, yet we typically treat it in sections and often neglect huge parts of it. One way to ensure that you are oiling it properly is by performing a daily self-massage. This can be done after your morning shower or bath or before you go to bed at night. According to ayurveda, oiling is actually cleansing and detoxifying. Full-body oiling lubricates the muscles and organs and helps loosen toxins from the areas of application. For example, oiling the stomach lubricates the intestines and gastrointestinal tract, while oiling tense shoulders can help loosen stiff muscles. Moistening the body and scalp also helps maintain good circulation by keeping the capillaries moist, especially if you use warming oils like sesame and avocado. People with cold hands and feet benefit from oiling them nightly.

Many ayurvedic remedies for psychological disorders caused by excess vata involve oiling the scalp. Due to the porousness of the hair follicles, the scalp is especially susceptible to deep absorption. Research has shown that when comparing hairless versus hairy mice, those with hair absorbed two to three times more product topically.

Makeup

Cosmetics are high-status items in our medicine cabinets. All women (and some men) know how a little makeup can make a huge difference in defining and enhancing natural features. But we often we overlook the chemicals in our makeup. We make sure our cleansers don't strip the acid mantle; our toners balance pH; and our creams are protective, soothing, nonclogging, and moisturizing. We spend hours (and fortunes) finding a regimen that best suits our skin's needs and conditions, and then we apply heavy liquid foundations, pore-clogging concealers, drying powders, and irritating rouges and shadows that undo all our hard work. Still, not many of us are willing to go makeup-free.

In recent years, more cosmetic lines have begun using natural ingredients (though some still contain cornstarch, which is natural but dehydrates the skin). Historically, these natural brands did not have the staying power or vibrancy of chemical ones, so many women opted for practicality over purity. But we no longer need to make this compromise, because the invention of mineral makeup has married clean ingredients with modern functionality.

MINERAL MAKEUP

My favorite cosmetic discovery has been mineral makeup. When I was going through the acne era of my life, I struggled to find a way to camouflage my skin without promoting more blemishes. I found mineral cosmetics to be invaluable; they allowed me to wear foundation without clogging my pores and provided SPF protection that helped my vulnerable skin after frantic overpeeling.

Mineral cosmetics are composed of 100 percent pressed or loose minerals—zinc, titanium, iron, and so on. They do not have dyes or perfumes, which are known to clog or irritate skin, and high-quality brands press the mineral powders with wax or oil, not chemicals. The minerals themselves are beneficial. Zinc is antibacterial and anti-inflammatory, and it provides natural sun protection. Mineral makeup is perfect for skin suffering from rosacea, acne, allergic reactions, and aging, since it is completely natural and soothes as it purifies. It also provides excellent coverage and is nondrying.

The first question my mature clients ask is, "Will the powder make me look old?" Regardless of ingredients or health benefits, if a product emphasizes lines and wrinkles, it's going in the garbage. Pure + simple mineral powders (and liquids) do not contain drying ingredients like talc or cornstarch, so they do not cake or look powdery or flaky. The light-reflecting properties of the minerals actually illuminates the skin while hiding imperfections, making the skin look younger.

The minerals provide all the pigment or color in this type of makeup, so chemical dyes are not required as they are with most cosmetics. Because it is pure pigment, the coverage is excellent. Finally, mineral makeup has amazing, long-lasting effects and is even water-resistant for up to forty minutes.

APPLICATION

Applying mineral makeup is easy! All you need is a clean brush or sponge. Apply it in layers, adding more opaqueness as desired and giving equal amounts of sun protection to your entire face.

The only prerequisite is that your skin must be moist or the makeup will not hold properly. Dry powder on dry skin does not adhere, and liquid foundations slide off oily skin throughout the day. For very dehydrated skin, I recommend applying a rich moisturizer or face oil before the mineral powder. Even someone with oily dehydrated skin can use a natural face oil as a base for powder makeup to create a seamless, finished look similar to that of a liquid foundation. Liquid mineral products are applied like any other liquid foundation.

It's not necessary to give up cosmetics and our desire to look polished when avoiding chemicals. While the term *au naturel* has traditionally meant to forgo makeup, today with safe, pure options such as mineral cosmetics, we can use makeup that is chemical free, provides SPF protection, and helps us achieve a more flawless finish to our skin.

Makeovers 101

Start with a clean base. Camouflaging imperfections to even skin tone makes an immediate difference. When you hide redness, blemishes, dark spots, and undereye circles, your features become more prominent. For example, less redness makes eye color more brilliant. If you don't need or want to use foundation all over a little dab of concealer will do the trick; however, a mineral base helps protect the skin. If you do use a full-coverage foundation, color-match it to the skin on your neck so you won't look like you're wearing a mask. If your neck and face are significantly different in color, pick an in-between shade to blend and even this out.

Tend to your brows. Eyebrows are my favorite part of a makeover and one of the most influential facial features. Darkening them gives the face more definition, while lightening them softens it. Always keep in mind that your brows frame your eyes. If they are too thick or dark, they will overpower and take attention away from the beauty of your eyes. If they are too light, you will look washed out. If you have mature skin, consider lifting the arch of your brows to help create a more youthful look. If you are unsure of how to groom them, consult an esthetician.

Use makeup to contour your face. As a woman of Asian decent, I have a flat nose and shallow features. While shallow features are beautiful, they can look swollen and shapeless. For this reason, I often contour my nose and cheekbones (especially on puffy-face days). Remember, dark makeup creates shadows and makes features recede, while light makeup highlights and brings features forward. I put dark color on the sides of my nose and light color on the tip.

I recommend camouflaging a turkey neck with dark contouring under the jawline and down the front of the throat. Of course, all makeup must be blended well for a natural, flawless look.

Give yourself some color. Using blush or a bronzer creates a healthy glow. After applying foundation, you may look unnatural without blush, because you have blocked out your natural cheek color. I have noticed that when I do television spots without heavy blush, I look more masculine, and my face appears flatter, because studio lights blanch the skin. When applying blush, start from the temples and blend down into the cheeks and along the cheekbone to contour and chisel your face. Applying soft color only on the apples of the cheeks emphasizes that area and softens the face.

Moisten your lips. Whatever else you do, always keep your lips moist. Even if you wear a matte lipstick to shift more attention to your eyes, do not use a product that sucks out moisture. Chapped lips are never in style. Glosses create a pouty, full-lipped look, whereas matte lipsticks flatten. If you do choose a more matte lipstick, I advise using a dab of face oil or a lip oil underneath to prevent flaky skin on the lips. Whichever you choose, the best products treat your lips while making you look great.

Match your lifestyle. Always choose cosmetics that are appropriate to the way you live. If you don't have time to reapply throughout the day, choose muted colors that won't start to look faded or "bleed." If you work in a professional environment, choose makeup that communicates your work persona. Light pastels can be youthful and soft, while darker, contrasting colors are more dramatic. Don't choose what is in vogue; go with what suits your coloring. Generally, people with a high degree of contrast in their natural coloring are best able to carry off dark, stark makeup. Dark-haired, fair-skinned people can wear wine reds and chocolate browns. Lighter, softer colors (and textures) are most suitable for people with little natural contrast. This can be dark-skin with dark hair, or light-skinned blondes. Redheads are usually low contrast as their hair coincides with skin that most often posseses pink undertones. Of course, these are general rules that can be broken to achieve a specific look.

These are only basic guidelines. Always use what makes you feel beautiful, comfortable, and attractive.

Five

Golden Rules for That Golden Glow

Now that you understand what the skin reveals about overall health and how it is affected by the body, mind, and emotions, we can focus on how to keep it beautiful using a long-term, holistic approach. The following are my "golden rules" for healthy, beautiful skin using modern science in conjunction with Eastern medicine.

Rule 1: Maintain Hydration

Like every living creature on this earth, human beings need hydration. This is essential, both externally and internally, to maintain health and proper cellular function. But people often confuse dry skin with dehydration. It is important to understand that dry skin refers to skin that lacks oil; dehydrated skin refers to skin that lacks water.

A lack of water causes fine lines. These are not laugh lines or deep wrinkles (which are caused by the breakdown or loss of collagen and elastin); they are easily minimized with the application of a water-rich skin care product. But if the skin is constantly dehydrated and depleted for a long time, other skin ailments or damage result that eventually translate into more severe signs of aging.

Although we associate moisture-depleted skin with age, we may not think of it as a cause of acne. Contrary to popular belief, it is often the drying of the skin that aggravates breakouts. When we look at acne from the standpoint of excess oil, we typically treat it with drying agents or "oil-free" products. Not only does this deplete and weaken the skin, leaving it vulnerable to acne infection, but it also disrupts the skin's oil flow. Instead of secreting on the skin surface, lubricating and protecting it, the sebum dries in the pores. This oil then hardens, resulting in clogged pores and encouraging the skin to produce even more oil.

Dehydrated skin not only clogs more easily, but it holds on to congestion, making extraction of pore buildup more difficult. Let's compare skin to soil. Weeds in moist earth are much easier to pull out than those in dry soil, which clings to the weeds and causes them to break off at the stem, leaving their roots intact. When doing extractions on dehydrated skin, it helps to use extra steam that allows the skin to hydrate and soften so buildup comes out easily. The steaming also reduces sensitivity and redness. The same analogy can be applied when waxing hair from dehydrated skin. To ensure removal of the hair roots, it is helpful to exfoliate and hydrate the skin a day before waxing. At Pure + simple, we actually oil the skin in preparation for waxing; not only does this facilitate root removal, but it also lessens inflammation. Think of how tight your skin feels when it lacks moisture. This stiffness causes skin redness from dilated and broken capillaries.

Specific skin ailments like eczema, rosacea, psoriasis, and dermatitis are also all aggravated by dehydration. Sometimes eczema worsens when oil is applied—despite this being a logical treatment for dry, flaky skin—because water is needed rather than oil, which increases heat (inflammation pitta). Allergic reactions and irritation can also be triggered or intensified by dehydration, which weakens the skin's immune system. None of these issues can be treated without first rehydrating the skin, which cannot heal if it does not have water. With the exception of fungus, almost all skin ailments require nourishment for rebuilding and regenerating.

To compound the problem, dehydrated skin is difficult to rehydrate because its absorption ability has been impaired. Let's use another earth/soil analogy. Hard, dry soil does not absorb water as successfully as soil that is moist, because the dryness creates a crustlike barrier and the water simply runs off. Many of my clients think their cream or lotion is too heavy because it does not penetrate well, yet their skin is dehydrated. The only way to overcome this is to be persistent with moisturizing products; the skin will gradually rebalance and be able to absorb properly again. So take a deep breath and keep using a superhydrating moisturizer. Exfoliation also helps because it sloughs away the accumulated layer of dry, dead skin cells and enables moisture to penetrate more deeply.

How to Hydrate from the Outside

Topical hydration provides the most immediate fix, and the right combination of water- and oil-based products is crucial, because layering moisturizers is the best way to increase water in the skin. Apply a serum to hydrate the skin, followed by a rich cream or facial oil to seal in the water.

But supplementing the skin with water is not the only way to boost moisture. Sluggish circulation also contributes to dehydration, because the blood transports nutrients to and wastes away from skin tissues. When this movement is disrupted, the health and vibrancy of the skin tissue is compromised. Good circulation also promotes collagen production, which helps the skin retain water and keeps it looking youthful and smooth. This is why the skin on the extremities dries out so easily—these limbs are furthest from the heart. Blood flow reaches them last, resulting in dry hands, cracked heels, and a flaky scalp (all of which are common during the dry winter months).

Choosing a stimulating serum or performing a short facial massage while applying skin care products helps improve circulation and also supports skin health and hydration. If your skin is sensitive, you cannot use intensely stimulating products, so start by incorporating gentle pressing movements into your application of facial products. As your skin becomes less dehydrated, it is also likely to become much less sensitive.

Avoiding harsh chemicals in skin care products is another moisture-increasing beauty practice. The use of depleting chemicals makes it nearly impossible for the skin to maintain moisture, so natural products without petroleum and sodium laurel sulfate must be part of any replenishing program. If you have taken all these measures and your skin remains dehydrated, it is time to examine internal factors.

Increasing Hydration from the Inside Out

The most obvious way to hydrate is by drinking water, yet some people drink plenty of water and are still dehydrated. As one of my clients joked, "I could drown in all the water I drink in a day, yet my skin still has no moisture!" Ayurveda attributes this condition to excess vata. Whether it is vata energy weakening the kidneys or increasing the rate of water evaporation, this air dosha can prevent internal water retention. Eating hydrating food, such as soups, stews, and vegetables with cellular fiber and high water content, is beneficial. This calms vata and forces water to move more slowly through the digestive system. It is also necessary to avoid dehydrating liquids, such as coffee and alcohol, and dehydrating foods, such as starches and dense meats.

Taking in oils and fats is another way to help hydrate. Oils hold water and lubricate the intestines, making it easier to eliminate. Clean bowels are important for hydration, because dry stools absorb water.

Pittas can also dehydrate despite high water consumption, because their intense internal heat dries up water. Dehydrated pittas often feel heat and dryness in the mouth and throat. Drinking slightly sweet liquids (from fruit and vegetable essences but not refined sugars) can cool pitta, as can drinking water with added minerals. This can be done by adding electrolyte tinctures or powders (sugar-free). Some people soak crystals in their water to "charge" it with minerals and healing energy. Pittas have difficulty digesting oils, which are heating, so monitor this carefully if you are taking in fats and oils to treat dehydration. Sometimes this will cause nausea, and fat intake should be decreased when this occurs.

Managing stress is another way to pacify vata and pitta to address dehydration. Stress is extremely dehydrating, not only because it increases pitta inflammation and vata nervousness, but also because it taxes the kidneys. The adrenal glands that secrete epinephrine (adrenaline) are located on top of the kidneys, so when you are stressed out, you overstimulate both the adrenal glands and the kidneys. Although relaxing spa treatments can be helpful, real lifestyle and mind-set changes are the long-term solution for this cause of dehydration.

Finally, as mentioned earlier, poor blood flow deprives the cells of nourishment and causes internal dehydration. This can be improved and increased through exercise and fast-paced massage, as well as by eating stimulating foods. Dark chocolate and warming spices are excellent foods for revving up circulation.

The Six Best Hydrating Ingredients

Here are some of the best ingredients for maintaining moisture in our skin. Look for these additives in your Skin Care to increase hydration.

1. *Collagen.* The skin's dermis layer is made up primarily of collagen fibers that swell with moisture and hold water when we are properly hydrated. As we get older, collagen production decreases, causing dehydration and signs of aging, so using skin care products containing collagen provides excellent supplementation and promotes skin hydration. While I have found collagen from fish to be most effective, a plant-derived version is also acceptable if you want to avoid animal products. "Plant-derived collagen" is not actually collagen, but it functions as a substitute and can still help with hydration and skin repair.

2. *Hyaluronic acid.* Hyaluronic acid is another substance that the body produces naturally. But unlike collagen, most skin care products and cosmetics that contain hyaluronic acid use a form derived from a plant source. Hyaluronic acid is extremely hydrating and is said to be able to hold up to one thousand times its own weight in water. Thus, skin care containing hyaluronic acid helps our skin retain water.

3. *Ceramides.* Ceramides are lipids found in the skin, but they can also come from plant sources. They are essential to maintaining our skin's barrier and therefore help keep the skin hydrated. Because dehydrated skin experiences both water loss and impeded barrier function, using skin care products with

ceramides are helpful for restoring hydration as well as preventing further loss of moisture.

4. *Aloe vera*. Aloe vera is full of water, and it is a wonderful anti-inflammatory and healing substance. It's widely used to treat sunburn, because it helps replenish and cool the skin. Aloe vera stimulates circulation slightly, so it is good at helping to regenerate skin tissue, but it can be aggravating for extremely sensitive skin. As an ingredient in skin care products, aloe vera is diluted to the point that it should not cause inflammation even in the most reactive skin types; however, using straight aloe vera juice or plant gel may cause redness for approximately one hour, after which it should subside. I recommend using straight aloe vera and products containing it if your skin is extremely dehydrated even if it does cause some redness, because the aggravation is only temporary and the benefits of this ingredient far outweigh its side effects. Remember, circulation also supports hydration.

5. *Algae*. The algae used in skin care formulations is seaweed, which lives in natural bodies of water, is full of cellular water, and contains numerous minerals. It helps the skin hold water and is excellent for fading scars and for antiaging. Algae is also slightly stimulating and can cause redness in people with excess pitta, which facilitates dilation of the blood vessels. Because it is so good for hydrating the skin, even people with rosacea should sample a product containing algae. Often, those with mild rosacea will not react to it. For everyone else, this subtle stimulation is excellent for maintaining proper blood flow in the skin.

6. *Sesame oil.* Sesame oil does not hydrate so much as it locks in moisture. It is a rich oil that reduces vata in the skin and seals in water; it evaporates from the skin's surface throughout the day. This oil also increases circulation, which may be too stimulating for pitta skin; this skin type should opt for coconut oil. But sesame oil is the best antidote for dryness and devitalization for both vatas and kaphas. It should be used on top of a water-rich serum.

Rule 2: Protect Yourself!

After ample hydration, good protection is key to healthy skin. All skin needs protection, and requirements differ based on genetics, geography, and exposure. Wind, cold, heat, dryness, sun, dirt, indoor climate control, and pollution all assault healthy skin, requiring balancing measures to restore and maintain beauty. Studies have shown that if the skin is protected from any type of injury, it has the ability to rebuild and regenerate itself even without rejuvenating or antiaging treatments (although they are still beneficial).

The type of protection needed depends on the environmental aggressors to which skin is exposed. As the seasons change, so must skin care regimens. Oil protection is necessary in winter, which is why you should change to richer creams during this season. A nourishing barrier helps heal and repair, as well as reduce vata, after you are exposed to dehydrating cold temperatures, harsh winds, and drying indoor heat; it also adds a layer of protection between your skin and the elements. In summer, you can use a lighter lotion, but protection is still essential. The focus of summertime protection shifts from dryness to ultraviolet (UV) damage. Because sun is probably the single most damaging environmental factor in promoting signs of aging, understanding proper sun care and how to measure protection is important. This next section discusses suncare in depth.

SUN PROTECTION

Sunscreen is probably the best-known skin protection. The sun has been cited as the primary source of hyperpigmentation, aging, and of course, skin cancer. The need for sunblock is indisputable, but so is the need for choosing the right one.

We require fifteen minutes of sun a day to obtain adequate vitamin D for healthy bones and teeth, but longer exposure (especially without proper protection) can damage skin's cells, causing premature aging. This occurs when UV rays penetrate the dermis, damaging collagen and elastin fibers. As a result, natural sunscreens are a new essential for proactive beauty care. For everyday use (when you are not spending too much time in the sun), apply them only on delicate areas—like the face, neck, and chest—so as not to impede vitamin D absorption. Sunblocks are available in lotions, sprays, and mineral makeup.

There are two types of sunscreens: natural blocks that use zinc and titanium to create a physical barrier against UV rays, and chemical blocks that neutralize and absorb UV rays into the skin's tissues. Chemical sunblocks are popular because it is easier to find them built into lotions and cosmetics. However, natural sunscreens are generally less toxic and less irritating, and they cause fewer allergic reactions.

The highest sun protection factor in most natural sunblocks is SPF 30. While our sun-fearing society may wish for higher numbers, high-level chemical sunscreens can actually heighten the likelihood of cancer because they contain proven carcinogens. Many sunscreen agents—such as octyl methoxycinnamate, octyl-dimethyl p-aminobenzoic acid (OD-PABA), benzophenone-3, homosalate (HMS) and 4-methyl-benzylidene camphor (4-MBC)—also upset the body's hormonal balance. In particular, a study conducted by the Institute of Pharmacology and Toxicology at the University of Zurich found that they have been shown to disrupt levels of estrogen, and traces have been found in breast milk. The higher the SPF, the more toxic the product, which is why some countries prohibit products making claims of an SPF higher than SPF 30. This is already the case in Australia.

Natural sunscreens sit on the skin's surface like a shield, so they do not need to be reapplied to stay effective. Chemical sunscreens need to be put on every one to two hours, because their ingredients become inactive. Researchers have found that people who are unaware of this suffer more sun damage because they don't reapply the product. Studies have also shown that even people who know they must reapply their sunscreen have a higher incidence of skin cancer because they spend more time in the sun and do not put the product on as often as necessary. Once erythema (redness from burning) begins, reapplication of sunscreen does not stop it. You must reapply the product *before* this happens and take breaks from the sun to let your skin cool. Remember, with each reapplication, more chemicals are absorbed into your body.

Natural sunblocks are a healthier option and provide a beauty benefit as well. Zinc is an anti-inflammatory that calms sensitive skin and an antibacterial that aids acne-prone skin. By contrast, many chemical sunscreens clog pores and irritate skin due to their toxic and petroleum content.

Measuring Sun Protection

The general misconception is that the higher a product's SPF, the more protection you get, but SPF only describes how long the sunscreen remains active. It represents the amount of time it takes for skin to burn multiplied by the SPF protection number. For example, if it takes five minutes to burn without sunscreen, using a product with an SPF of 15 will extend the time to seventy-five minutes (15 × 5).

Actually, the difference in filtration of UV rays between SPF 15 and SPF 30 is minute—96 percent and 98 percent, respectively. Sun-conscious countries like Australia have banned sunscreens with SPFs higher than 30, which can mislead consumers into thinking they are safer than they are. The high concentration of chemicals in such products also causes free radicals, which leads to premature aging of the skin.

Ray Type	Effects of Overexposure
UVA	•Skin damage • Premature aging • Skin cancer
UVB	• Erythema (redness from burning)
UVC	• Skin cancer

Protection for Prevention

Many people wait until they have a problem before they fix it, whether it is a major health condition, an issue in their personal life, or a skin ailment. While they may be able to remedy the problem, they can never reverse the situation back to its original state, and the same is true for the skin and body. Sun damage can fade, but skin cells are permanently affected. Acne can be cleared, but scars can linger.

The people with the most beautiful skin are those who have been forward-thinking enough to prevent the damage. People with sensitive skin should take precautions against rosacea; fair-skinned people should use extra protection against sun damage; and everyone should engage in antiaging therapies.

Furthermore, corrective treatments are not always without side effects. Dangerous surgeries and peels can not only end up making skin look artificial, but they can damage cells, nerves, and tissues. Hyperpigmentation, scarring, and permanent sensitivity are only some of the lasting effects of many treatments.

It is easy to let a problem progress through lack of attention, but you should love and care for yourself before an emergency or a trauma occurs. Listen to your body and care enough about yourself to be proactive. Remember, you only get one body and one complexion in this life. With protection in mind, you can truly honor your body as the sacred vessel it is.

Rule 3: Be Gentle

We live in a culture that encourages us to be tough on ourselves as a measure of success. "Beauty is pain," "no pain, no gain," "go big or go home" are all sayings that reflect how much we link results with harsh and extreme methods.

This not only affects our self-esteem, but it crosses over into our grooming habits. We often want to overwash, overscrub, and overdry our skin to rid ourselves of dirt, blemishes, and the like. Having worked abroad, I have found that North Americans especially love to overexfoliate, creating oil imbalances, dehydration, sensitivities, and irritation. But stripping the skin does not yield the best results. It is a very delicate organ, and mistreating it actually compromises its barrier. When we are not gentle in our care, we disrupt the skin's acid mantle—the surface coating of sebum that is made up of fatty acids, salts, and lactic acid. Since this mantle creates a protective layer against bacteria, overcleansing and drying it decreases its resilience, immunity, and general health. Even for people with acne, I prescribe a gentle regimen, because stripping the skin further provokes the production of excess oil. Gentleness is also important to prevent or modify signs of aging, because inflammation or trauma to skin tissue produces free radicals. These molecules damage skin cells and lead to fine lines, wrinkles, and poor texture.

Pampering Principles for the Skin

The first and most important way to pamper your skin is to avoid chemical ingredients in your skin care products. Chemical dyes, perfumes, and detergents aggravate and damage the skin and create imbalance. As mentioned throughout this book, sodium laurel sulfate is especially detrimental; it is so caustic that it is often used to degrease heavy machinery.

But even natural ingredients can be drying. Use the more astringent hydrosols (the water components of steam-distilled herbs), essential oils, and herbs only when necessary. For example, tea tree oil is too harsh unless you are trying to kill an acute infection. Even if you have blemish-prone skin, opt for something more gentle like lavender oil or hydrosol as a daily antiseptic. If you have ultrasensitive skin, it is also wise to avoid high concentrations of peppermint or rosemary oil (looking at the product's list of ingredients—those with the highest concentrations are listed first). When using purifying plants and herbs in your facial regimen, use hydrosols, which are much more diluted than plant oils. But again, if your skin feels dry or tight after application, do not use them for an extended period.

Simply avoiding products that overstimulate or irritate is another way of being gentle. Even though stimulating circulation is important, you must not induce redness or reactions. Staying clear of allergens is immensely important, since the more stress you put on your skin, the less healthy it becomes—just as eating foods you are sensitive to taxes your immune system. The antidote is to use skin care items made with soothing, nurturing ingredients. Anti-inflammatories such as German chamomile, sandalwood, coconut oil, calendula, rosewater, aloe vera, oat beta glucan, and zinc oxide all help comfort the skin and decrease heat. They also pacify pitta. You can take many of them orally to get the same effects.

Finally, use a soft touch when caring for your skin. Do not rub it abrasively; be gentle and loving. Even when towel-drying, pat your skin instead of wiping it. Try to avoid picking your skin, which can cause bruising, bleeding, and scabbing. See an esthetician for extractions, and make sure he or she is gentle; blackheads should never be forced out, and only those that are easy to remove should be extracted.

All these practices will also help maintain a youthful appearance and avoid tissue damage, dehydration, and free radicals.

Rule 4: Calm Down

Both modern medicine and holistic practices agree that stress is detrimental to our health. Awareness of this helps us understand that our emotions also affect our body and skin. It is surprising how beneficial simply relaxing and grounding yourself can be to your complexion. Healthy individuals have a glow that naturally draws others to them, and being well rested is a vital part of that radiance. But it's impossible to get adequate rest if you're under chronic stress, and the combination of the two depletes your whole immune system. Stress is incredibly taxing, and in the long term, it leads to premature signs of aging, dehydration, water retention, inflammation, and weight gain. Stress makes you more susceptible to dry skin and fine lines, which in turn contributes to oil imbalance, acne, poor absorption, sensitivity, hyperpigmentation, allergic reactions, dullness, and clogged pores.

One reason for all this havoc is that stress-related fatigue depletes the adrenal glands, which leads to dehydration. As discussed at the beginning of this chapter, hydration is the single most important factor for the health of the skin, the immune system, and the body as a whole. Some health practitioners believe the adrenals are so important that they must be treated before any other healing can occur. Because they regulate stress and energy levels, improving their function helps all of the other organs work better. The adrenal glands are located above the kidneys (which control the retention and release of water), and they secrete adrenaline when the body is under stress. Adrenaline protects us by providing extra energy to combat danger; however, when the adrenals are overstimulated for a long time, they cause the kidneys to be overstimulated as well, and the body loses water.

Stress-induced constipation can also cause dehydration. When you are under a lot of stress, the anxiety often causes tension in the muscles. You may think this type of muscular tension is limited to the neck and shoulders, but many people actually carry stress in the abdominal area. This affects the intestinal muscles, causing them to tense up and making elimination more difficult. Constipation is dehydrating because blocked bowels absorb water. Diagnosing stress-related dehydration from the skin is easy, because it is not cured by applying creams or drinking liquid. For this reason, facials are dually beneficial; they treat the skin and promote relaxation. At Pure + simple, our Lymphomaniac

Facial includes a stomach massage along with a lymphatic drainage massage.

From an ayurvedic view, all these conditions are indicative of vata aggravation. Both the kidneys and the colon are governed by this dosha, and because of the delicate, unstable quality of air, the resulting symptoms of dehydration, weight loss, and memory loss have a vata quality. Vata imbalance can also lead to dysfunction in the other doshas.

One example is kapha water retention. Because the body becomes accustomed to losing water when under continual stress, it begins to store excess fluid to prevent depletion, leading to a kapha imbalance. This creates heaviness in the body along with puffiness around the eyes and face. But this extra fluid is not distributed in a healthy way nor does it nourish tissues as normally metabolized water does. Instead, this edema (retained fluid) collects turbid water in the legs, face, and lymphatic system. People often mistake this swelling for weight gain, but fat reduction is unnecessary; water retention is treated by eliminating kapha foods, emptying the bowels, rehydrating the body, and most important, lowering stress levels.

Stress can also lead to a pitta imbalance, causing a craving for calories, especially from sugar. Ambitious, perfectionistic, high-pitta people crave sweets because a sweet taste cools their heat. An overactive mind stresses the body and creates a desire for calories. This is why people who spend a lot of time on computers are often addicted to candy bars: sugar satiates the brain. Too much mental stimulation causes a rise in cortisol, which the adrenals create along with adrenaline. Cortisol is produced to soothe inflammation in stressful situations. According to Leo Galland, MD, author of *The Fat Resistance Diet,* constant secretions of cortisol caused by too much stress are harmful and lead to weight gain around the stomach area, creating a "spare tire" around the midsection.

Stress creates inflammation, resulting in the accumulation of excess cortisol and pitta. This is why type A personalities often exhibit flushed skin. Repressed anger and other stressors create unreleased internal heat, which increases the heart rate and dilates the capillaries. Burst and broken capillaries are more of a cardiovascular disorder than a skin condition. Blushing from embarrassment and flushing from strenuous exercise are symptoms of acute stress that translate into inflammation. This is why stress reduction is a major part of managing rosacea; it is also why many people have more reactive skin and are prone to breakouts, rashes, and eczema during times of stress. Dermatologists often prescribe hydrocortisone cream to treat redness and reactions (because cortisol helps diminish inflammation). As described in chapter 1, these creams are harmful over the long term by making users dependent on external cortisone and compromising their immune response. But oversecretion of adrenaline and cortisol does not just produce excess fat and dehydration; it also leads to hormonal imbalance.

When you are under stress, your body makes adrenaline production a priority, neglecting the production of other hormones and throwing your whole system out of balance. For example, underproduction of the hormone progesterone adversely affects menstruation and fertility. Hormonal acne can be traced to the production of excess testosterone, which stress also encourages. Infertility, dysmenorrhea (painful periods), and amenorrhea (the absence of periods) are prevalent health issues of the modern age, reinforcing how a stressful lifestyle can really affect health. The body is a holistic system, and the hormonal system illustrates this.

THE DISCIPLINE OF RELAXATION

A commitment to relaxation is a commitment to self-respect and self-love. We often neglect this commitment in order to tend to our families and careers; we even feel guilty when we make ourselves a priority.

While letting go and allowing yourself to focus on relaxing takes great discipline and can seem even more difficult than exhausting yourself with actual tasks, it is essential to your health. Being a stress martyr doesn't do you or those around you any good, and it can cause long-term exhaustion. You are not only most beautiful when you are at peace, but you are also in the most positive state to be the best possible parent, spouse, friend, and team member.

When I talk about stress reduction, I always remember when I gave a composed, middle-aged woman her very first facial. After I cleansed her skin, we had a nice chat about its condition. She told me she needed a simple regimen because she was the mother of three boys and had hardly any time to cleanse her face, morning or night. During the extensive neck and shoulder massage that I do as part of the treatment, she started to weep. "I don't remember the last time I was this relaxed," she said. Though I didn't know if her tears were of joy or sadness over her self-neglect, releasing her emotions allowed her to let go and fully express how stressful her life was.

Whatever it is that pulls at you, you need to let go sometimes and put yourself first. Long-term stress sacrifices your health, your ability to perform personally and professionally, your happiness and naturally, your appearance.

Simple Tools for Stress Reduction

When you find that everything stresses you out, it is an indication that you are not as healthy as you could be. Your mental and emotional selves cannot cope with the extra load. When your body is weakened by imbalance, the small speed bumps in your day become major hills. I am a fairly high-strung individual, and my relationship with stress used to be so strong that I began to see my stress-prone behavior as an illustration of my commitment to my work and relationships. But my sense of urgency for each daily task did not display how much I cared; it really demonstrated the lack of commitment I had to my own health. It also made me more erratic instead of more effective. When I realized this and began to look for ways to let go a bit, I found that stress reduction isn't about a few breathing or visualization exercises, it is a mind-set and a lifestyle choice that must be woven into our daily routine.

The first and most important tool for staying calm is regularity. Having a routine is extremely relaxing, because it takes the guesswork out of your plans and makes going through your day more like dancing to beautiful, rhythmic choreography. The most challenging but most beneficial routine is eating regular meals. The schedule of a business owner can be unpredictable, and I found that when and what I ate mirrored this lack of predictability and caused irregular digestion. This in turn made me less effective. When your digestion or other bodily functions feel uncomfortable, it is difficult to feel strong and grounded. Eating at the same time each day is not only excellent for the digestion, it also allows your body to know when it will be nourished and how to distribute energy evenly. This helps you maintain a constant blood sugar level throughout the day, without falling prey to synthetic energy boosters like caffeine or refined sugars.

Regularity in your physical fitness regimen also helps cut down on stress. Whether it is rising early each morning to do yoga or taking an after-dinner walk, building exercise into your day expends nervous energy and keeps your body fit. When your circulation is strong, your joints supple, and your muscles robust, your body is healthy, agile, and comfortable. You can effortlessly move through your life and this sense of physical harmony contributes to a sense of well-being. A consistent exercise schedule allows you to put aside special time to rejuvenate your body, reflect, and perhaps enter a meditation-like state. Our physical health is very much a part of our emotional health. Although the West often views the psychological and physical selves as separate, with different theories and different doctors for each, ayurveda connects them to each other and to the environment.

Spending time outdoors naturally instills a sense of peace. This is understood in ayurveda; a respect for nature is deeply embedded into its philosophy. Both sunbathing (to accumulate warmth) and moonbathing (to cool the constitution) are healing therapies to rebalance the vikruti. In yoga, a Tree or Mountain Pose is a simple homage to the natural world. Stress is purged when we make time to be in nature. Trees and plants absorb carbon dioxide and emit oxygen through photosynthesis; when I am surrounded by lush plant life, I feel like I am drinking in nourishing, oxygenated air and can really exhale. Even if you just go to a nearby park or meditate in your backyard, honoring your connection to the earth every day is important—not only to remind yourself of its gifts and beauty, but also to help you remain balanced and take a break from the treadmill of modern society.

Meditation is another way to separate yourself from the busyness of your life. It is the act of uncluttering your mind and focusing on the present moment. While it may seem as easy as sitting in Lotus Position and closing your eyes, meditation takes an incredible amount of discipline. When you meditate, you let go of all of your inner chatter and your self-imposed obligations. But this is very difficult, and there are many different methods and schools of thought on how to meditate. Some people use visualization, some chant mantras, and some focus their concentration on something tangible such as a candle flame to center their attention. Whatever way you decide to try, all forms of meditation aim to pull you from the chaos and distraction of the active world and help you achieve clarity and contemplative awareness. Setting time aside to meditate regularly lets you realize the true triviality of your everyday stressors and conflicts.

PROPER SLEEP

Sleep is invaluable to your well-being. When you are tired, it is difficult to cope with stressful situations. I used to joke that sleep was a commodity I wished I could bottle and sell because it is so important, yet many of us do not get deep sleep or proper amounts of it.

During sleep the skin and body regenerate, so when you do not get good sleep, you become prone to acne and inflammatory breakouts and accelerate aging. This overworks and weakens your adrenals and kidneys, which causes dehydration of the organs and skin. Overproduction of adrenaline occurs when you do not fall asleep during kapha time (in the evening before 10 P.M.) and provides an unnatural source of energy. This often results in insomnia, producing an unwelcome "second wind" even when you are exhausted. Without ample sleep, the body finds it difficult to heal the stress and damage the day has put on your skin and tissues. Whatever energy you have goes into maintenance, and when all your reserves are used, you crash, becoming vulnerable to disease. But besides the detriment that a lack of sleep causes your overall health, it also has a direct effect on your complexion.

During a seminar I attended on antiaging, a cosmetic research scientist presented the direct effects of poor sleep on the skin. The speaker and his team had studied "clock genes," genes found within the cells of the body that allow synchronization of cellular activity with the circadian cycle. I found this especially interesting because the circadian cycle or clock is much the same concept as vata, pitta, and kapha time. Both state that we experience different rhythms throughout the day that dictate temperature and energy fluctuations, and the times when these fluctuations occur also correspond.

The speaker said that each cell has its own "clock," and this is governed by a part of the brain called the suprachiasmatic nucleus. Found in the hypothalamus (or "the master clock"), the suprachiasmatic nucleus interprets "night" in relation to the levels of light to which we are exposed as well as the amount of food and activity we experience. The hypothalamus also carries communication between the nervous system and the endocrine system, which relates to the observation that our well-lit modern society contributes to the widespread occurrence of hormonal imbalance (an idea first introduced to me by Dr. Vasant Lad).

The speaker and his team also observed how skin tissue repaired at night because clock genes induce protective antioxidants. They found that when clock genes were synchronized with the circadian clock, it actually enhanced the skin's resistance to UV damage and enabled the cells to restore themselves. But they also found that clock genes were unable to synchronize after subjects had acquired a sunburn, because this UV damage caused DNA damage.

I always knew that sleep was important to skin health as a by-product of helping the immune system and body stay in balance, but what I learned at the seminar demonstrated the definite cause-and-effect relationship between a sleep-deprived, overstressed lifestyle and skin aging.

Given how important sleep is, you should know what to do when you have trouble falling or staying asleep. As someone who has often wrestled with these issues, I have discovered a few simple yet crucial techniques to overcome insomnia and interrupted sleep. While sleeping pills and natural sleep-inducing supplements are effective, they do not change or address the root issue. Similar to chronic skin ailments, lifestyle problems such as these are an expression of imbalance in your doshic energy.

Take Your Time Getting Ready for Bed: Trouble sleeping is an indication of vata excess because the mind is overactive. This is why it is important to slowly unwind well before you actually try to sleep, gradually comforting and mitigating your vata energy. If you have chronic problems sleeping, start your nighttime routine with a warm bath. Submerging the body in heated water pacifies vata's cold, dry qualities. Follow this with massaging your body from head to toe with sesame oil. Both the relaxing act of self-massage and the use of sesame oil, which is a vata remedy, help calm nervous energy. Even though I recommend taking time preparing for bed, this does not mean you should go to bed late after a long evening regimen. In fact, it is important to try to fall sleep by 10 P.M. at the latest, since this is still kapha time, when you are at your most grounded. It is when you enter your pitta and vata times at night that it becomes difficult to fall asleep.

Limit Media Exposure at Night: Vata governs the sensory organs, and bright lights from computer monitors or television screens stimulate vata and make your mind unnaturally active. The same goes for exposure to backlit clocks and streetlights that shine into your bedroom. While it may be tempting to work on your computer well into the evening or watch your favorite late-night television program, these habits are terrible for getting a good night's sleep. If you feel restless in the evening, settle into bed with a good book instead—just avoid reading suspense or other anxiety-inducing literature.

Don't Eat Late at Night: Eating stimulates digestive activity, which also keeps you awake. Eat at least two or three hours before bed to ensure proper sleep and good digestion. Eating late at night is hard on the heart and also makes it difficult for the body to relax and prepare for rest.

Increase Your Water Intake: While the inability to fall asleep is a vata issue, waking up late at night is a pitta issue. This is often triggered by internal dehydration and low water intake. When your body is overheated and in need of cooling hydration, it prompts high heat that wakes you up. Sometimes drinking water immediately upon waking can help you fall back asleep quickly. And to prevent interrupted sleep, increase your water intake throughout the day.

Exercise Early in the Day: Exercise is great for reducing stress. This is especially important for vatas who tend to be cerebral and often forget to reconnect with their physical body. But exercising too late at night is stimulating and inhibits proper sleep. Schedule exercise in the morning or during the day, and if you feel you have a vata imbalance, make your workouts slower and more grounding. Fast-paced cardio training increases vata, whereas hatha yoga and resistance training help mitigate this doshic energy.

Ayurvedic Antistress Treatments

Groundedness is a cornerstone of health, according to ayurveda, since it is only through stillness that we can become enlightened. Because out-of-balance vata energy is the source of anxiety, nervousness, and worry, antistress treatments should be used to pacify this dosha. Vata is often the first dosha to lose balance (in excess), and it facilitates other imbalances and disease, so there are many ayurvedic treatments that specifically target vata.

One of the best ways to reduce vata is with oil. Whether taking it orally or applying it topically, the nurturing properties of oil help with the drying depletion that vata creates. Kapha's best vehicle for the absorption of medicines is traditional ayurvedic wine; pitta's best medium is ghee; and vata's is sesame oil. Herbal infusions added to wines, ghees, and oils help these ingredients permeate into the organs associated with each dosha as well as their tissues (Kapha: fat, Pitta: blood, Vata: nerve endings and bone tissue). While plain sesame oil is excellent for treating vata, especially in the treatments outlined here, sesame oil infused with herbs is a more focused remedy for excess vata. Ashwagandha sesame oil helps build muscle that has been weakened, while sesame oil infused with shatavari helps restore compromised reproductive health. You can purchase both ashwagandha and shatavari from health food stores and retailers selling ayurvedic oils; you may even find vata blends with a mixture of these herbs in sesame oil. Using them in traditional ayurvedic treatments is a wonderful, calming addition to your personal care regimen.

Another traditional ayurvedic treatment is *abhyanga*, which is a type of massage that manipulates the marma points (energetic points), disperses the lymphatic fluid, and promotes relaxation. It uses liberal amounts of dosha-specific oils to treat imbalances. It is usually performed by two therapists who coordinate and synchronize their movements, massaging the body together. This treatment is excellent, because it swathes your skin's nerve endings in oil and also focuses your attention on your body's sense of touch. This is why I find massage so sacred; it creates tranquillity in both the body and the mind. It reminds you to care for your body and not live too much in your mind. If you do not have access to a place that offers abhyanga, doing self-massage while applying sesame oil to your entire body with long, soft strokes can offer similar benefits.

Shirobasti is a treatment in which a tubelike leather "cap" is placed on the head, and oil is poured through the top to saturate the scalp. This sits for approximately an hour. Shirobasti treats many psychological disorders as well as headaches and insomnia. In extreme situations, the head may be shaved so the oil can have direct contact with the scalp; when the hair is left intact, this treatment also deeply nourishes the hair shaft and follicles.

Shirodhara is one of the most popular and widely available ayurvedic treatments in spas and ayurvedic clinics. It involves dripping oil onto the "third eye" and the scalp from a metal vessel with a small opening in the bottom. The third eye is found between the eyebrows and is said to be the gateway to consciousness. This treatment settles the nervous system, releasing serotonin and calming the mind. It can done for varying lengths of time (usually an hour to an hour and a half), depending on a person's doshic tendencies. While kaphas have the patience to experience Shirodhara for long periods of time, pittas can usually last for only a moderate span of time, and vatas get restless and want to stop after only a short interval. It is most beneficial for vatas (and of course those with vata imbalance), so even if the client gets antsy, a treatment of at least twenty to thirty minutes is advisable. If you cannot find a practitioner who can perform Shirobasti or Shirodhara, oil your own head with sesame oil. Drench your scalp in oil, separating the hair into sections and really working the oil into the scalp. You do not want the oil to be soaked up by the hair itself, because the contact with and absorption through the scalp is what is truly therapeutic. The oil should be left in overnight and washed out in the morning.

Rule 5: Decongest

Decongesting the skin and body means keeping them clear of buildup and stagnation. Whether we refer to it as detoxifying, cleansing, shedding, decongesting, exfoliating, eliminating, or clearing heat, purging accumulation is a natural part of life. The body maintains itself by constantly ridding itself of toxins and wastes to make way for rebuilding and regrowth. We cannot survive without this cycle of renewal.

Detoxification and elimination of waste helps us stay healthy, not only physically, but also mentally and emotionally. Purging negative feelings and past experiences, along with excess ego, is important to our well-being. People often consider their thoughts to be separate from their body, but blockages in the mental self manifest in the physical self. When we see how stress causes hair loss or embarrassment translates into a blush, it confirms how directly our mental state influences how we look. Knowing this, it is important to highlight how detoxifying the mind can help keep us healthy and mentally acute. Even the act of throwing away possessions and clearing out closet clutter can be therapeutic.

North Americans have recently become obsessed with physical detoxification. Fasting, flushing, and colon therapy are now so mainstream that they are almost glamorous. But if you detox, you must maintain balance and do so gently. Recognize that too much elimination can be depleting to your internal organs, and overwashing and overexfoliating can be counterproductive to your skin's health. It is essential not to get too preoccupied or obsessive about cleansing programs. Nonetheless, decongestion is an important part of every skin regimen, and when done properly, it is the best way to attain a bright, vibrant, clear complexion.

DECONGESTING THE SKIN

When the pores are clear, the skin can absorb properly, sebum flows freely, and a smooth texture is maintained. This is achieved when skin is being hydrated and protected with healthy, natural moisturizers. When the pores get congested despite proper care, it is not a topical issue but one of environment or internal imbalance; stress, changes in weather, improper diet and poor digestion, illness, medication, and doshic dysfunction can all cause buildup. That being said, people who live in urban settings deal with invasive damage caused by daily exposure to smog and pollution, creating pore congestion that is nearly impossible to clear without extra help.

The following are a number of excellent ways to decongest your skin.

Extraction: The quickest and most effective way to unclog pores is through extraction. Squeezing and picking should always be done during a facial treatment, after the pores have been softened with hydrating serums, peels, and steam or hot towels. It is best to have extractions done by an experienced professional who knows how to proceed without bruising, scarring, or spreading bacteria. This is especially important if you have sensitive or problem skin.

After extraction, the skin must be purified with a natural antiseptic (such as witch hazel) and the pores tightened with a treatment mask. When done correctly, extractions keep the pores clean, small, and fine.

Exfoliation: Exfoliation is great for preventing congestion. Removing dead skin promotes cell turnover, oxygenates the skin, and improves circulation. Technological advances have produced many forms of exfoliation to fit each skin's goals and needs, making choosing the right product easier than ever.

Scrubs are the most widely known exfoliants. They contain a granular, abrasive agent to physically slough dead cells from the surface of the skin. In the desert, where there is little water, some people simply use sand as a cleanser and exfoliant, because it keeps the skin polished and therefore clean. Know what exfoliating agent is in any product you use, because some ingredients can scratch and damage the skin (see chapter 4). The gentlest scrubbing agents are jojoba pearls (wax beads).

Chemical peels and newer, more intense peels containing agents—such as alpha hydroxy acid (AHA), beta hydroxy acid (BHA), glycolic acid, lactic acid, or one of many fruit acids—do not require manual scrubbing. Despite being labeled "chemical," they may use naturally derived acids to digest surface skin cells. Pure + simple uses corn-derived lactic acid and natural fruit acids in our skin-refining products. The base of a peel is important because natural ingredients are gentler and penetrate more effectively. But apply these peels with caution. Frequent use makes the skin more vulnerable to UV rays, which causes sensitivity and irritation and can lead to hyperpigmentation. Monitor the percentage level of the agent carefully. When I had acne, I was given 70 percent glycolic peels by a dermatologist. This increased my sensitivity and damaged my skin. All peels wound the skin to promote regeneration, but with chemical peels, you have less control over the depth of exfoliation and the amount of irritation caused.

While both scrubs and chemical peels can be done at a spa or clinic or as an at-home treatment, some deeper exfoliation treatments can only be done properly by a professional. Microdermabrasion uses a specialized machine to buff, abrade, and "sandblast" the skin. It is often referred to as a controlled peeling, because the technician (esthetician) can adjust the depth of the peel by monitoring the skin throughout the treatment. A series of microdermabrasion treatments is an excellent antiaging tool, because it helps promote circulation, cell turnover, and collagen production.

There are a few varieties of microdermabrasion. My personal preference is sea-salt microdermabrasion, because it uses all-natural salt crystals instead of the traditional aluminum crystals. Sea salt is much better for the skin. Not only does the salt disinfect, but it dissolves in water, unlike aluminum crystals that can leave residue lasting for up to two weeks. I have worked extensively with both forms of microdermabrasion and have found that the sea-salt variety offers a deeper peel with less irritation and yields better results.

Steaming: Steaming is a fantastic, noninvasive way to sweat out impurities. It opens the pores and promotes circulation. Also, when herbs and essential oils are added to the steam, the skin absorbs them on a deeper level because of the dilation of the pores.

Steaming must be done twice a week or more to really see results. This is a great option for pus-filled and cystic acne skin where extractions risk spreading bacteria, as well as for sensitive skin that is easily marked or scarred. It is an easy practice to do at home, and it has been very effective for clarifying many of my clients' complexions.

Here are some simple instructions on how to do an at-home steam treatment:

1. Bring water to a boil in any kitchen pot.
2. Remove the pot from the heat and add herbs or essential oils (if available) that correspond to your skin type and ailments. For example, if you have kapha skin with blackheads and blemishes, use peppermint tea bags or sage essential oil, which are both purifying and have antimicrobial properties. Sensitive pitta skin can use chamomile tea bags or calendula essential oil, as they are soothing and have calming properties. Vata skin, which needs antiaging help, benefits from ginseng tea, tulsi (holy basil), or ginger oil, which promote circulation and rejuvenation.
3. Hold your face approximately six inches above the steaming pot and drape a towel over your head to trap the steam.
4. Sit under this tent for up to five minutes. If you are prone to redness, do it for only three minutes, but if you do not have sensitive skin, you can steam for the full five minutes. Since perspiration makes you lose water, replenish your skin afterward with either a moisturizing mask or a replenishing serum and moisturizer.

This treatment not only decongests the skin, but it is a common treatment for opening the sinuses.

Oiling and Oil Massage: Using oils to detoxify the pores may seem unconventional, but as mentioned earlier, oils regulate oil production and actually have cleansing properties. Massaging your complexion with pure vegetable oils will help loosen deep-seated and embedded buildup in the skin. This was revealed to me many years ago while I was doing a facial on an acne sufferer in her late twenties who was very dehydrated yet was petrified of using moisturizer for fear of breaking out. She had some pustules, but her main problem was blackheads, which covered her chest, back, shoulders, and face. During the steaming portion of the facial, I performed an extensive oil massage to make her extractions easier and prevent redness. However, as I worked, the hardened oils in her pores began to loosen, and the blackheads popped out like little corks. I had to wipe off my hands and reapply more oil several times! It was a remarkable experience, and needless to say, the client was not afraid to apply oil to her skin after the treatment.

A Gentle Ayurvedic Protocol for Daily Decongestion

Cleansing the body is not something to be done intensively once in a while; it should be done daily in a more gentle way. This section describes some traditional ayurvedic therapies that can easily be incorporated into your schedule to prevent a buildup of congestion and help your system stay healthy.

Using a Neti Pot: Breath is sacred in ayurveda, which is why keeping the nasal passages clear is considered essential to good health. The lungs and respiratory system are one avenue of elimination, and when they are congested, it inhibits detoxification as well as full oxygenation. Remember, oxygen helps feed cells and repair tissues. Using a neti pot every day is one way to keep your airways clean. It is a small pot with a long spout through which you pour a concoction of salted water into your nasal passages. This concoction is made by filling up the neti pot with purified water then adding half a teaspoon of sea salt. Then you tilt your head sideways, pour the water into the top nostril, and let it run out the other side. I do this each morning during allergy season or anytime my nasal passages are congested. It helps me feel alert and rejuvenated in the morning and alleviates facial puffiness.

Using Nasya: Nasya is the administration of medicines through the nasal passages. Such medicines primarily come in powder or oil form. Sometimes herbal decoctions and juices are also used.

Powder dries up dampness in the respiratory system, while oil lubricates. Nasya can be done daily and is another form of maintaining proper respiration. Most often, daily nasya involves tipping your head back and dripping the oil into each nostril with an eye dropper. Nasya oil is easy to find, and while there are many different oils, those found on the market are usually tridoshic and fit for all body types. Nasya oil lubricates and cleanses the nasal passages. It often dislodges phlegm so you can spit it out. While the water from a neti pot cleanses, nasya oil treats dryness. Do not follow either treatment immediately with the other; use them on alternating days or use one treatment in the morning and the other at night.

Powder nasya is excellent for kaphas who have issues with mucus and water retention, because it reduces this moisture. It does require a pumplike sniffer contraption that may be hard to find. Salt inhalers are a more common option. An ayurvedic salt inhaler is based on the same idea as using nasya powder, but the former is a little more gentle. You use a ceramic container like a sippy cup that is filled with salt; inhale the salty air through your mouth and exhale it through your nose. This clarifies the respiratory system and alleviates asthma, chronic coughs, and other related ailments. There are no contraindications. Breathing through a salt inhaler for fifteen to twenty minutes per day is ideal for purifying the lungs.

Scraping the Tongue: The tongue is a mirror to your overall health, and it is said that a healthy-looking tongue should look like a rose petal. Unhealthy bodies express themselves through this organ. A white coating on the tongue indicates dampness and kapha excess within; a yellow coating demonstrates heat and pitta excess; and a black coating or cracks in the tongue indicate excess vata, as well as vata-related shoulder and back pain.

You want to eliminate toxins on the tongue by scraping it each morning. Scraping before brushing means you will not push the toxins into the gums or gradually ingest them as you swallow. It also ensures that bacteria is removed from the oral cavity and helps reduce bad breath. Copper tongue scrapers are best for excess kapha and are warming and naturally antibacterial; silver tongue scrapers cool and have antimicrobial properties, which is best for pitta. Stainless steel tongue scrapers are tridoshic.

Gargling with Oil: Ayurveda recommends swishing the mouth with oil each morning. You can use anywhere from two tablespoons to a cup of sesame oil and swish for a minimum of fifteen minutes. Sesame oil is antibacterial and antifungal, as well as nourishing. The oil cleanses and draws out toxins in the mouth and tongue, which is beneficial for total body health.

From a strictly oral perspective, this also cleanses and strengthens the gums and keeps the teeth beautiful and strong. Always spit the oil out after gargling, as it contains toxins and possibly parasites. While the sensation is odd at first, your mouth will feel clean and refreshed after swishing it with oil.

Oiling the Ears: Continuing ayurveda's love affair with oil, ear oiling is another practice that can be done every day. The ears and sense of hearing are governed by vata, so inserting a few drops of sesame oil into each ear helps prevent dryness, protects the ear canal, and helps treat auditory issues such as loss of hearing and ringing in the ears. Vata governing the ear area and sense of hearing is also why those with high vata or people in the vata stage of life lose their hearing.

Oiling also loosens excess wax and prevents wax buildup. According to ayurveda, earwax is excreted from muscle tissue and produced during muscle metabolism, and when the overall muscle tone and quality is compromised, it can result in excessive earwax.

While this treatment may not seem directly related to beauty, it is only when all of your systems work properly that you are in balance and therefore beautiful. Keeping the passages of the ears moist and decongested mitigates the vata component of this sensory organ, and you are more open to awareness when all of your senses are intact.

Taking Triphala: As described in chapter 2, Triphala is a tridoshic powdered laxative of three dried fruits (amalaki, bibhitaki, and haritaki). It can be taken nightly by the half teaspoon with warm water, or upon waking first thing in the morning. Triphala has even been compared to a mother, as it is so caring and restorative for the body and its functions. Dr. Vasant Lad has joked, "Forget Visa cards. Triphala: Don't leave home without it." Taking this detoxifying mixture helps purify the tissues and maintain clear, glowing skin.

Now that you are familiar with the tools and methods of maintaining balance for the skin, it is time to discuss more specific beauty ailments. The next section explains how to rescue your skin holistically from chronic conditions such as acne, rosacea, and signs of aging. The chapters will help you self-diagnose and treat these persistent skin disorders, both topically and through balancing your internal health.

Part Three

BEAUTY 9-1-1

Six

Acne: The Journey to Clarity

Acne, zits, pimples, pustules, blemishes. Whatever we call them, we detest them, and in this age of high stress, pollution, and processed foods, they're widespread. For some people, acne may be a minor annoyance, but for others, it undermines self-image and lowers self-esteem. "I couldn't even look people in the eye," one client told me. Such people are easy prey for the false promises given by makers of "deep-pore cleansers" and "oil-free creams." I was one of those people.

The problem is that many of us are misinformed. When I had acne, several doctors and estheticians told me that my blemishes had nothing to do with my diet or my general physical and emotional state; however, until these were addressed, I saw no changes in my skin. Many dermatologists and skin care professionals concentrate solely on topical pimple formation as a basis for treating acne. While it may seem logical to identify and eliminate the factors that cause a blemish, this does not provide long-term results. From this perspective, blemishes are simply clogged pores that have become infected and inflamed, sometimes turning them into pustules. This is why many acne solutions focus on reducing sebum, minimizing blackheads (through peeling), and using antibacterial agents. But why do some people develop clogged pores while others do not? Why do some comedones turn into acne, while others simply remain congested pores for years?

The answer lies in the fact that acne is both an internal and an external problem. It is an expression of imbalance that cannot be overcome by looking only at the blemishes and their formation. Acne is complex, with a multitude of causes, and is most often aggravated by many factors at the same time. It is a highly unpredictable condition, with varying levels of severity, making it impossible to give a blanket solution to all acne sufferers, which is often the approach of conventional skin care professionals.

As I have described in other chapters, in my struggle with acne, I actually made my skin worse through my own short-sightedness and naïveté. What began as a small imbalance caused by poor skin care choices paired with hormonal changes turned into a decade-long skin problem. Desperate to clear up my complexion, I dried out my skin (which depleted its defenses), accumulated heat and inflammation from my own stress and frustration, and finally damaged and weakened my internal health by using powerful antibiotics. If I had known then what I know today, I would have simply taken a deep breath and recognized my acne as a signal to examine my overall health. Armed with the information in this chapter, I would have been able to make more informed decisions based not on emotions but on the consciousness and awareness of my own body's systems.

Internal and External Causes of Acne

To understand the best approach to use when trying to clear up your acne, you must first identify the causative factors. While some blemishes are aggravated by imbalances on the skin surface, others come from internal health issues. It's important to distinguish between them, because when you treat the real causes of your acne, the improvements to your skin will be both dramatic and long term.

Clogged Pores

Clogged pores are a precursor of acne, because the encapsulation of a pore is what traps bacteria beneath the skin. Excess oil is the commonly blamed culprit for acne; therefore, it is generally believed that stripping the skin of its oils will prevent and clear up blemishes. But this does not actually cure acne. Instead, it causes dehydration, which is the root cause of overproduction of sebaceous oil, which initiates a vicious cycle. Congested skin is often caused by stripping away oil. The absence of oil makes the body produce more oil to compensate in an effort to create balance. This extra sebum is thicker than normal to try to protect the skin. So the result of using oil-free products or not using a moisturizer creates an even bigger oil problem.

Oily skin is the most beautiful and healthiest type, if properly maintained, and it should never be stripped. It needs gentle care and lots of hydration to maintain clarity so that sebum does not dry and solidify in the pores and create blackheads. Dehydration is actually the most common cause of acne (and also contributes to scarring). While sebum overproduction may set the stage for clogged pores and blemishes, acne does not occur without dehydration. A lack of water in the skin is what dries out facial oil so it sits in the pores instead of flowing across the skin surface to protect and lubricate. Breakouts often occur during the seasonal change from summer to fall or in a move to a less humid environment. Even skin types with little sebaceous activity accumulate blackheads and congestion when they are dehydrated.

The skin must be hydrated from both the inside and the outside. As people who have acne become more hydrated, not only does their skin clear up, but it becomes moister, less sensitive, and less irritated. With many of my acne clients, improved hydration and a decrease in sensitivity also allows me to do more thorough extractions and skin purification without the risk of scarring. Eating lots of fresh vegetables and drinking at least two liters of water a day cleanses your system and hydrates your cells. Avoid dehydrating foods and activities such as caffeine, alcohol, and smoking, which are dehydrating and taxing to the liver. While going to sleep early and avoiding alcohol is ideal, a topical boost of moisture can lessen the effects of bad habits. If you are getting to sleep too late or indulging in a glass of good wine, use a rich moisturizer or face oil before going to bed. This deeply feeds your skin overnight and minimizes the consequences of skin dehydration.

Proper skin care is a necessity when combating dehydration (and therefore clogged pores). Since you cannot control how your body absorbs and disperses the water you ingest, applying moisturizers to your skin is an essential support and the most direct way to fight superficial dehydration. Nourishing, oil-based products also help seal water in, preventing the evaporation of precious hydration.

As we have discussed previously in this book, the concept of fighting acne with oil may be surprising to many acne sufferers. It is often difficult for acne-prone people to take this approach because they are so used to avoiding oil; many of my first-time acne clients have been using a gel moisturizer or none at all. But once they begin to use pure oils on their skin and see an improvement, they become oil enthusiasts. One of my most devoted clients came to me when he began breaking out in his thirties. He was frustrated because he had never had problem skin before, even as a teenager. Although skeptical, he began using a facial oil as his nighttime moisturizer. His skin became so much clearer and less congested that he happily used the oil regularly and switched to an oily textured milk cleanser as well.

It is important to emphasize that I am talking about using only natural vegetable oils, not petrochemical-based moisturizers or mineral oil. Natural skin care is essential for maintaining hydrated, acne-free skin.

Harsh chemical cleansing agents dehydrate the skin, and as explained earlier, petroleum-based products sit on the skin, inhibiting moisture absorption and clogging the pores. Sometimes the use of chemical-based skin care products is even the initial cause of breakouts. In such cases, the switch to a natural regimen helps diminish acne on its own.

When making this kind of switch, think beyond your basic skin care routine to include your sunblock and cosmetics. Many acne sufferers depend on cosmetics to hide their blemishes, worsening the problem. Even if you use proper, high-quality natural skin care products, the clogging effect of commercial makeup can prevent the skin from clearing fully. When you ensure that everything you put on your skin is made from pure ingredients, overcome your fear of oil, and increase your body's and skin's hydration, you eliminate the occurrence of congested pores, which is fundamental to achieving clear, blemish-free skin.

HEAT AND INFLAMMATION

Pimples and blemishes are forms of inflammation. Therefore, anything that increases inflammation, whether it is topical or internal, also triggers breakouts in acne-prone skin.

Direct, topical heat such as sun exposure can prompt acne breakouts. Abundant sun exposure can cause this in a pitta constitution because this heat pushes out toxins. The sun also stimulates the sebaceous glands while drying out the skin. Excess exposure resulting in sunburn traumatizes the skin and taxes its immunity. This creates a lot of heat in the skin's layers and damages them, leaving the skin vulnerable to more blemishes.

Another topical heat factor is the use of products that stimulate circulation. While blood flow is excellent for feeding skin cells, too much circulation in acne-prone skin leads to more blemishes. Ingredients like ginseng, rosehip oil, and vitamin C are great for rejuvenation and repair, making them effective for healing scars, but they also aggravate breakouts in acne-prone skin. Use them either as spot treatments for scarring or after your skin has normalized and stopped breaking out.

Although external heat increases inflammation on the skin, internal heat is closer to the root cause of acne. Avoiding topical heat is fairly easy to do, but internal heat is a result of excess pitta, and the body attempts to purge this hot energy. According to ayurveda, the first thing to examine in cases of inflamed acne is the circulatory system. Because pitta governs the blood, and the blood feeds the skin directly, acne is known to be a *rakta dhatu* (blood) disorder. In this case, the blood is considered "dirty," loaded with pitta heat and other toxins such as kapha dampness.

Cleansing the blood is key to clarifying the skin. Blood-purifying herbs are also pitta reducers, and a knowledgeable ayurvedic physician or naturopathic doctor can help you choose which ones are best suited to your constitution. If you would like to start with something subtle and simple, incorporating turmeric in your daily meals is an excellent way to pacify pitta and gently clean the blood. This spice is tridoshic, so it is a good choice for all body types.

Turmeric supports good digestion, decreases excess stomach acid, calms inflamed skin, and removes heat from the liver. One of my clients, who broke out in a terrible heat rash with pustules, found that taking turmeric capsules in conjunction with daily meditation and a pitta-pacifying diet was immensely soothing. Her breakout was so severe that I thought it would take two weeks to ease and would leave scars, but with the help of the turmeric, her skin improved dramatically within days and remained unmarked afterward. A common dose of turmeric is two to four capsules with meals, but if you decide to use it this way rather than as a flavoring spice, consult a health practitioner to determine the best amount and consumption method for your constitution and situation.

Eating a pitta-reducing diet is also important for treating inflamed acne. Although many acne sufferers know that food affects their skin on a daily basis, there is the misconception that simply eating less junk and fast food is sufficient. In actuality, you need foods that calm inflammation. According to ayurveda, this means avoiding circulation-stimulating foods and liquids such as coffee and hot spices like cayenne, black pepper, and chili. Eating water-rich foods also fights fire, so cucumbers, melons, and sprouts are good for pacifying pitta. But when incorporating hydrating fruits and vegetables into your diet, you must stay away from those that are acid forming, such as grapefruit, sour cherries, plums, radishes, and tomatoes. One client who followed these recommendations admitted, "I was a bit skeptical. How could tomatoes be bad for me? These restrictions seem so specific, but it makes sense now, and my skin is much clearer."

Sweet grains such as white basmati rice and barley are also excellent, because they are bland and counteract spicy foods. Dairy and wheat are also pitta balancing for this reason, but avoid these kapha-forming foods if you have wet, pus-filled blemishes.

The liver is another organ to assess when dealing with acne, because it stores heat. Chronic acne (especially adult acne) is an indication of a liver imbalance, and even the best skin care products cannot heal this. The liver is the body's filtration system; if it is overheated and overworked, it does not absorb or filter properly, and excess waste spills into other areas. Because the skin is the largest organ of detoxification, toxins that cannot be filtered and eliminated will end up here. According to ayurveda, the liver is closely related to the emotion of anger, making someone with a weak liver prone to irritability. This is important because all acne is related to the pitta dosha, and pitta behaviors increase the presence of heat in the liver and skin (and vice versa).

While eating an anti-inflammatory diet is excellent for reducing heat, so is cooling the mind. Pittas often have difficulty calming down, so rest is important. Sleep helps to regenerate and detoxify the liver, and according to natural body rhythms, the liver usually detoxifies from 1 A.M. to 3 A.M. This makes sleep during these hours extremely necessary to the health of the liver and, because of its filtration role, that of the rest of the body. The liver filters many hormones, so when it is not functioning properly, this influences the endocrine system. Instead of being cleansing and eliminating excess hormones from the body, a weak liver can lead to a buildup of them. This gives way to other hormonal issues, because much of hormone production is based on the body's estimation of how much it has. This can cause an imbalance in the excessive, improperly filtered hormone as well as the regulation of others. As we've discussed, all systems in the body are interconnected, and hormones play a huge part in the treatment of acne.

Hormones

Hormonal imbalances are a common cause of breakouts, evidenced by the fact that many women get flare-ups around the time of menstruation and during pregnancy, and men and women experience skin problems during puberty and times of hormonal change midlife. In the ayurvedic view, hormonal change causes an excess of internal heat, and again, the result is acne. Common hormonal imbalances also create this excess; for example, heightened testosterone both heats and increases sebum, while excess estrogen creates inflammation. Out-of-balance hormones are a sign of out-of-balance doshic energies. It is important to understand this and not assume that you cannot change your hormonal patterns or that hormone supplements or replacement therapy is the only treatment.

Sometimes excess pitta that affects the liver is the root cause, and liver cleansing helps normalize hormones. In other cases, kapha excess causes polycystic ovary syndrome (PCOS), a syndrome in which cysts are found on the ovaries and that is often linked to excess male hormones as well as imbalances in estrogen production. In this case, avoiding kapha foods and taking herbs aimed at reducing cysts (such as neem) can be effective. Even many Western doctors recommend that PCOS patients avoid starches and high-glucose foods, which is an essential part of a kapha-balancing diet.

With the help of a knowledgeable alternative health practitioner or physician, you can heal the real cause of a hormonal imbalance and treat your endocrine system naturally.

CONSTIPATION

As mentioned earlier, the skin is an organ of elimination. This means that when the body is backed up with too much waste, it tries to expel toxins through the complexion. One obvious sign of constipation is an abundance of blackheads along the jawline and lower cheeks. Chronic constipation is a major cause in moderate to severe acne, so regular bowel evacuation is necessary for clearing up the skin.

One client, with whom I'd been working for three years, had such congested skin that she wouldn't go anywhere without makeup. When I did extractions, it seemed as if almost every pore was clogged. In most facials, I allot fifteen minutes or so for extractions, but hers took me well over an hour. When she returned for follow-up treatments, every pore would again be full of dried sebum. We tried many different approaches, but her skin would clear up for only a few weeks at a time before she suffered yet another severe breakout. I couldn't understand why we could never stabilize her. She was a holistic nutrition student with an excellent diet; she drank three liters of water a day and exercised regularly. We tried to track her stress levels and did frequent facials with only minimal results. Finally, I asked her how many times a day she eliminated, stating that twice was ideal.

"Really? I'm lucky if I have a bowel movement every two or three days!" she exclaimed.

With such a buildup of toxicity in her body, it was no wonder she was eliminating through her skin. I had assumed she had regular bowel movements because she was so educated about food and the body, and I was shocked to hear how constipated she was.

I recommended that she take a tincture of milk thistle for her liver and drink half a cup of aloe vera juice with water twice a day. Aloe vera cools pitta and works as a mild laxative. I also prescribed a fiber-based laxative. Amazingly, after about a month, her skin looked smooth and clear. I was sure she must have resorted to taking strong antibiotics or birth control pills, but she announced with a smile, "I've only done what you told me to do, and I'm not even wearing makeup. You changed my life!"

This illustrates how the body always attempts to balance itself and stay healthy. Remember, if you do not release toxins through the bowels, they will come out in other ways, such as through your skin.

Stress

Stress taxes the whole body, lowering its immune system, causing it to dehydrate, leaving it defenseless against bacteria and infection, and decreasing its ability to regenerate. Constant anxiety causes the production of adrenaline, which unbalances the endocrine system. Many people experience major breakouts in stressful situations because they create internal inflammation; this is also why some people experience stress-related hives, eczema, and rashes.

Another reason distress leads to acne is because it causes tension in the abdomen. According to ayurveda, relaxation of this area is important for proper elimination and digestion. While you may not notice that you are holding stress in this area, it results in poor digestion (often causing gas and bloating) as well as constipation. This is one reason that stomach breathing during yoga practice is so beneficial. (See chapter 5 for other tips to reduce stress.)

While stress may simply seem to be a catalyst for other acne triggers, it is so common and so important that it needs to be mentioned separately. The first step in treating stress is to identify that you are actually under pressure. Sometimes it is such a regular part of life that you forget your mind and body are under strain. In some ways, the presence of clogged pores and pimples is a good reminder to analyze your behavior and reassess your lifestyle choices.

Conventional Solutions and Why They Don't Work

As we have discussed, acne is not strictly a topical skin ailment, which is why a superficial approach cannot cure it. It takes sensitivity to your body's needs, a respect for your health, and a lot of patience. Unfortunately, many people feel patience is a luxury they can't afford.

Many panicked teenagers seek the advice of dermatologists at the first sight of blemishes. The popular solution is to dry the skin with salicylic acid and benzoyl peroxide or to peel it with harsh retinol creams. This only worsens the problem by unbalancing and depleting the skin, causing more blemishes. Stripping also leaves the skin more susceptible to infection and, therefore, acne. Because acne rarely goes away with these methods alone, the next step is usually a more invasive one: antibiotics, birth control pills, and Accutane. Many people take antibiotics for teenage acne; although their skin clears up, their complexion becomes blotchy, dry, flaky, and sensitive, and they experience side effects such as nausea and a weakened immune system. When they stop taking the medication, since their root health issues have not been addressed, their acne often returns—even worse that it originally was. Many of my clients come to me with their skin in terrible condition after deciding to stop their antibiotics or birth control pills (which were taken as an acne treatment rather than a contraceptive).

Drugs provide only a short-term solution and leave dreadful after-effects. Antibiotics do a lot of damage, because they dehydrate the internal organs and cause photosensitivity (vulnerability to the sun). Hydration is imperative for waste elimination, so the medication ends up intensifying acne in the long run. Like a dried-up river, the system cannot flow and flush itself when it's dehydrated. Even topical detoxification in the form of extractions becomes difficult, because dried out skin holds on to pore congestion.

Antibiotics also weaken the liver. As we discussed earlier, ayurveda says that adult acne is usually liver-related, so when acne sufferers take antibiotics, they run the risk of further damaging their already dysfunctional liver for temporary results. This increases heat and agitates internal inflammation, which purges fiercely when they discontinue the drugs. As a side effect, the heat also creates skin sensitivity and promotes broken capillaries and reactive skin.

Birth control pills are another quick-fix solution. Artificially altering hormone levels is harmful to both the skin and overall health, and the result of going off the medication is often severe acne. Again, because the root cause of the acne was not addressed, it simply lies dormant and accumulates more internal inflammation. The body has so much excess hormone it attempts to detoxify when usage is stopped that it results in a huge skin breakout. It usually takes about a year to completely rebalance the skin.

Accutane, otherwise known as isotretinoin, has become popular in recent years because it is very effective, and after an initially painful period of severe breakouts, it clears acne up well. Accutane is made up of high-dosage vitamin A and works by drying up all of the oil glands. But this is harmful to the skin long term, causes premature aging, and compromises overall heath. Unfortunately, its clarifying results are also not permanent. This treatment is especially popular among men, possibly because their acne becomes severe so quickly due to their higher testosterone levels and because of their lack of education about skin care.

Accutane is extremely hard on the body, and common side effects include dry skin, constipation, vaginal dryness, inflammation of the liver, possible genetic damage, and dehydration of the internal organs. Accutane has also been linked to more than thirteen hundred psychiatric side effects such as severe depression, and according to the U.S. Food and Drug Administration, it has been cited as the cause of more than sixty-six suicides. Even one round of this medication can be incredibly damaging to internal organs, the immune system, and emotional health and well-being.

Affected Parts of the Face and What They Mean

If acne is product-related, it generally appears all over the face, as that's where skin care products are applied. But when pimples are isolated in specific areas, they indicate an internal problem. Referring back to the face maps in chapter 2, you can see the relationship between different parts of the face and the internal organs.

According to ayurveda, vata governs the top of the face, pitta controls the middle (undereyes to upper lip), and kapha rules the lower part. When these doshas are out of balance, acne will gather in the corresponding areas. For example, allergy breakouts on the upper cheeks relate to the lungs. People who quit smoking may also break out here, because inhaling cigarette smoke causes the body to create and retain a lot of internal heat, and pitta toxins purge as the body starts to detoxify.

Excess kapha manifests on the chin. This is often is due to an imbalance in the reproductive organs, so women coming off birth control pills may experience breakouts here (often in the form of cystic acne). The jawline is also kapha territory, and boil-like breakouts show up when this dosha's energy trait of retention builds up. Kapha imbalance, in the form of candida and sluggish bowel elimination, also promotes dampness in the body and translates to acne in the lower face.

The forehead, with its thin vata qualities, breaks out when there is dysfunction with the air dosha. Vata is related to the colon, so ensuring that this organ is hydrated and evacuated helps clear up blemishes in this facial area. Vata also governs movement, so dysfunction and stagnation in the lymphatic system (congested vata) can cause clogged pores on the forehead. Lastly, a hyperactive mind is the result of high vata and leads to dehydration—a major cause of acne—in this area of the face.

The affected sections of the face and the type of acne indicate what is happening inside the body. While unsightly, acne may actually be beneficial, because it indicates that the body is purging toxins rather than holding them where they could lead to more serious damage. Blemishes can be an early warning sign of illness and organ dysfunction.

Types of Acne

The type of blemishes you experience indicates more about their causative factors. Knowing the different categories of acne helps you determine the qualities of your internal imbalance and facilitate proper treatment.

In my practice, clients complain most about milia (whiteheads) and comedones (blackheads), which are also called "noninflammatory acne." Whiteheads occur when sebum and bacteria are trapped beneath the skin's surface. They may be virtually invisible or appear as white, hard-to-extract bumps. Blackheads occur when the trapped sebum and bacteria are partially open to the skin's surface. When the melanin in the skin oxidizes, they become black in color. Blackheads can be precursors to blemishes, or they may simply remain as they are—clogged pores.

Papules and pustules are more severe forms of acne. These pitta-type blemishes are categorized as "inflammatory acne." Papules appear as red bumps; they do not come to a head and are usually smaller than pustules. Pustules are red, inflamed bumps with a white, pus-filled head; what we generally think of as pimples. While the presence of pus indicates a bacterial infection related to pitta, an abundance of fluid is associated with kapha, so pustules have both a pitta and kapha quality to them and indicate imbalances of both of these doshas.

Cystic acne (also known as "blind pimples") consists of large, tender-to-the-touch pimples. They have no white head and are deeply seated in the dermis layer of the skin. These long-lasting blemishes lie beneath the skin and are sometimes invisible. They embody the kapha qualities of wetness and accumulation. Sometimes, cystic acne does show redness and inflammation, which indicates some pitta imbalance as well.

Cystic acne stays for a long time, so relief often involves having to remove the pimples by pricking them with a sterilized needle and extracting the fluid. Only a professional should do this, because cystic acne scars easily.

Holistic Solutions for Vata, Pitta, and Kapha Acne

The process of overcoming acne should not be like fighting a war, but most people view the condition as an enemy. When they see a pimple on their face, they want to eliminate it, extract it, and dry it out. If it feels like you against your acne, you're going on the belief that acne is a topical and external problem rather than the expression of an internal imbalance.

After years of thinking and behaving like some sort of pimple warrior in a losing battle, I realized that I needed to be kinder to my skin. When I began to look at my acne as my body making a cry for help, I started making it healthier as opposed to damaging and depleting it. Only then was my skin able to heal itself and my complexion improved. Stopping my use of harsh peels and detergents was only the first step. Using my breakouts—their size, qualities, placement, and timing—to diagnose which of my doshas were out of balance was what truly cleared up my acne. This newfound attitude toward my skin and body made my overall health much better, and not only was my complexion pimple-free, but it took on a radiance I had not seen in years.

Vata Acne

As explained previously, vata acne consists of noninflammatory blackheads and whiteheads. These blemishes result from vata depletion, dryness, and dehydration, and they often cluster in areas with thinner skin (the forehead and temples). They multiply and worsen when you attempt to clear them up with conventional astringent acne products, creating more whiteheads and dried out, clogged pores. While these blemishes can be bearable, with their small deposits of sebum and dirt, they lead to larger, more inflamed pimples if the imbalance is not treated.

Topically, the first thing to do with vata blemishes is to lubricate the skin. Start with a face oil or rich cream. A neutral oil like jojoba is good because of its medium weight and similarity to the skin's own sebum. I have never had a client break out from or react to pure jojoba, making it a safe option even if you are wary of introducing oil into your regimen. This usually yields significant results in a matter of weeks. Underneath, use a natural serum whose high water content will increase hydration, quenching thirsty skin and allowing it to heal and regenerate.

Besides reducing vata through moisture, you need to exfoliate this type of acne. If your skin type is also vata, the exfoliation must be done carefully because the skin is so thin. A gentle scrub two to three times per week helps immensely, especially when you steam the skin for five minutes beforehand. If your acne exhibits qualities of doshas besides vata and pustules are present, a peel is better so you do not break open blemishes and spread bacteria.

Sometimes topical measures alone can diminish vata acne, but more often you need to address your internal health as well. You need to nourish the skin through diet and eat hydrating, moistening foods that are heavy, sweet, warm, and wet—such as vegetable soups and moist rice dishes—to pacify vata (see the food chart on p. 41). Vata blemishes may also be caused by drying toxins within the colon (a vata organ), so always consider constipation. Water-rich, warm foods help soften stools and allow for better elimination. Being liberal with oils, essential fatty acids, and water intake is also important, as is the incorporation of heating spices like ginger and cumin. They help stimulate the digestive system, which is excellent if you have excess vata and are prone to poor, irregular digestion and bowel evacuation.

If you do not find relief in dietary changes alone and feel you need professional assistance with dry, constipated bowels, seek the expertise of an ayurvedic physician or practitioner. One therapy they may employ, which is excellent for reducing vata energy as well as lubricating and cleansing the colon, is an oil enema (basti). Oil, whether applied to your face, ingested through your diet, or inserted into your intestines, is incredible for vata pacification.

Finally, you must address vata acne by managing vata emotions. Anxiety, worry, and stress all tax the kidneys, dehydrate the body, and create tension in the digestive tract. Lack of or interrupted sleep also increases vata and puts you in a state of mind that contributes to nervous feelings. Refer back to the "Calm Down" section in chapter 5 for tips on how to manage both stress and insomnia.

Pitta Acne

Pitta embodies inflammation, and the blemishes it produces are red, angry, and inflamed. They can occur all over the face or primarily in the cheek area. Some pitta pimples contain pus, while others (papules) simply look like red bumps.

Pitta acne demands some antibacterial measures, but addressing inflammation (both inside and out) is more important to eliminating these breakouts. Skin with pitta acne must be soothed, and all cleansers, toners, and moisturizers must be free of drying, astringent ingredients such as alcohol. Ingredients like coconut oil, chamomile, witch hazel, and melissa (lemon balm) are excellent, because they are naturally antiseptic and calming.

Pitta acne also needs hydration, and the use of serum and oil assists in healing as well as skin purification. Serums containing aloe vera are especially fitting because of this plant's water content and cooling action. Coconut oil is best for pitta skin types and pitta acne, and its light texture does not aggravate heat like other, more fatty oils do.

Pustules (which have both pitta and kapha properties) can be particularly unsightly, as they have a white cap of pus on top of a reddened blemish. But even though you want to clear them up, do not exfoliate them. Scrubs can make these pimples burst and spread bacteria all over the skin, infecting previously acne-free areas. Nonabrasive peels are an option, but because they can also increase inflammation, use them with caution. The more kapha (wet and full of pus) blemishes are, the more effective nonabrasive exfoliants are. These types of peels are antikapha; they are slightly drying and break up fluid accumulation in the skin. But if you have more papules than pustules, you will want to mitigate pitta and avoid too much peeling. Peels can be applied as spot treatments as necessary or all over your face when you first begin your healing regimen. Nonetheless, you should incorporate nonabrasive exfoliants into your skin care regimen only as advised by an esthetician.

Peels such as sea-salt microdermabrasion can be performed by a professional who is trained to control the depth and vigor of the exfoliation and to avoid areas that are better left untreated. The antibacterial properties of the natural salt used in this procedure help to clarify the skin underneath the surface of dry skin cells.

Extracting pustules when they are "ready" is the fastest way to heal them. But it is difficult for untrained individuals to determine when this is; people get emotional over acne and often try to perform extractions prematurely and too roughly. This can lead to scarring and the recurrence of the pustule. If you cannot see a professional, try applying a drying clay or mud as an overnight spot treatment. This helps dry and draw out the blemish so you don't need to extract it.

Balancing pitta internally is also important. Eating cooling foods such as raw, watery vegetables and steamed bitter greens helps reduce this impaired dosha. Natural medicines such as amalaki and turmeric also help by balancing heat and can be taken in tea, capsule, or powder form or used fresh in food. Amalaki is a small fruit that is cooling and packed with antioxidants; turmeric root is an antibacterial, antiviral, and anti-inflammatory herb that is also a staple of many Asian cuisines. It is rare to find either of them fresh; they are most often available only as dry powder that can be used as tea. To make tea, add half a teaspoon of herbal powder to hot water, steep for ten minutes, then strain. Both amalaki and turmeric can be found in capsule form from a number of ayurvedic supplement companies (see "Ayurvedic Herbs and Supplements" in the resources section of this book).

Water consumption is also essential to this type of acne, because proper hydration reduces internal heat. Adding various supplements to your drinking water can help with its absorption. I put a few tablespoons of liquid chlorophyll, aloe vera, or kelp extract in my one-liter reusable water bottle to help me fight dehydration and excess fire dosha throughout the day. Liquid chlorophyll is an extract of the green pigment from plants. It is incredibly alkalizing, making it excellent for reducing inflammation and pacifying pitta. If you prefer to use aloe vera, the juice makes the best additive. Some formulas are made from the whole leaf, while others are made from the inner fillet. The latter is preferable because it is more of an anti-inflammatory than the former. Kelp extract is a liquid concentrate. Kelp not only contains a number of nourishing minerals, but it also helps you retain water and hydration, so it's an ideal additive to your daily water supply. All three of these ingredients are common staples found in health food stores.

Water additives and a cooling diet also help restore a weak liver, which according to ayurveda, stores heat and causes acne by preventing toxins from being filtered out of the body. As mentioned earlier, pitta governs the liver, and when this organ is not working properly, it can lead to hormonal imbalance—and hormonal acne. In this situation, people with pitta constitutions must do a monthly liver cleanse. There are many different types of liver cleanses, but a simple and traditional ayurvedic cleanse consists of taking one to two tablespoons of castor oil once a month. This expels dry stool from the bowels, gets rid of the heat that has built up in the small intestine, and cleans the liver. An ayurvedic physician can determine if this is the best treatment for each individual.

Finally, ridding yourself of this acne type involves keeping pitta emotions in check. Anger, irritability, and self-pressure all cause imbalance and are common emotions experienced by teenagers and menopausal women, along with pitta acne. Breathing exercises can be particularly helpful, and yoga practice offers healing exercises called *pranayama* (controlled breath). In the next chapter, we will discuss step-by-step breath work that helps control aggravated pitta and therefore is effective for diminishing stress-related blemishes. By alleviating your internal fire, you can stop your skin from being the avenue of heat dispersion and get rid of pitta acne.

Kapha Acne

Like the kapha dosha, kapha acne is all about accumulation, heaviness, storage, and dampness. Blemishes triggered by kapha imbalance are large, deep, full of fluid, and clear up very slowly. Classic kapha acne is cystic and hard to treat topically, because it does not occur in the superficial epidermis layer of the skin. These cysts are usually found on the chin or along the jawline, and according to ayurveda, they are most often related to yeast in the body or an imbalance in the reproductive organs.

As noted earlier, acne is a known symptom of polycystic ovary syndrome. The formation of cysts on the ovaries often contributes to cystic blemishes, and one of my clients discovered she had PCOS thanks to her pursuit of clearer skin. From an ayurvedic perspective, PCOS is commonly an expression of too much kapha, though this is not always the cause. It is a complex health disorder, so consulting a natural health practitioner who has a good understanding of the endocrine system is important.

One topical treatment for cystic acne is arnica lotion or tincture. Arnica is readily available in natural health food stores. It helps drain the fluid from a cyst by promoting circulation and breaking up the stagnation of the kapha dosha. If you have this type of acne, you must try to stay hydrated, because dry skin can accumulate dead skin cells and lead to ingrown hairs on the face and body. These can easily become infected, causing boil-like cystic breakouts. Apply both a serum and a lotion morning and night. Products that include algae (usually listed as "algae" or "algae extract") as one of their ingredients are an excellent choice, because they subtly promote circulation and help the skin hold water.

For kapha acne, you need to eat a kapha-reducing diet, which means avoiding oily foods, dairy, sugar, shellfish, bananas, and heavy starches. Purifying foods such as kale, fennel, burdock root, and mustard greens are excellent for balancing excess kapha. Apples are especially good for this dosha, as they are vata in quality and help dry up kapha wetness. This also helps reduce pustules, which are blemishes that have both pitta and kapha influences.

The herb neem is fantastic for clearing up cystic acne. Neem reduces kapha and pitta, and it has both calming and purifying properties. I have prescribed it to many clients in capsule form, with two capsules taken with lunch and dinner, but neem can also be taken as a powder or tea. Many of my clients saw their cysts disappear completely after they started taking this herb, while others found that it simply helped heal their cysts more quickly. You can apply neem oil topically, and it is good for many skin rashes and even topical parasites. Neem powder can be mixed with water to make a paste, which you can use as a mask treatment for both cystic acne and pitta acne. For a list of retailers that sell neem, refer to the resources section of this book.

Stimulation and lymphatic movement are imperative for balancing kapha excess. Exercise and vigorous massage both help move kapha accumulation and purge mucus. Both are good for preventing the formation of cystic acne, as well as cysts in other areas of the body.

Kapha skin tends toward kapha acne and clogged pores (which are due to dryness and excess vata). This is because oily skin types are so often advised to use skin care products that dry out the skin and remove oil from its surface. If you have this type of skin, you need to use a deep peel (only kapha skin can stand up to this treatment); follow exfoliation with a rich moisturizer or oil. This is the same treatment as for vata acne, only with the addition of the deep peel.

This chapter has given some examples of how acne can become worse when you treat it with methods that actually work against your natural constitution. When you do not embrace the beauty of your doshas, you end up creating problems and actually aggravating your imbalances. Because the skin is a reflection of overall health, working toward groundedness and internal nourishment leads to a smooth, clear, and healthy complexion.

Seven

Seeing Red: Sensitive Skin, Rosacea, and Eczema

Sensitive skin types have high pitta and react to internal or external stimulation with redness, dilated capillaries, and dermatitis. Whether it is simple flushing or an inflamed rash induced by an allergic reaction, the root cause of sensitivity is stimulation of the cardiovascular system. But although all these symptoms indicate sensitive skin, all sensitive skin is not the same and should not be treated in the same way. Rosacea, eczema, and allergic skin are all inflammation-based ailments, but they are very different conditions and must therefore be pacified by very different care. Rosacea is primarily characterized by dilated capillaries (blood vessels) in the skin and is rooted in an overly stimulated circulatory system, whereas eczema can manifest as an itchy rash or simply flaky skin.

Labeling skin "allergic" does not necessarily mean that it is prone to flushing and redness; it means skin is reactive to various or specific stimuli that cause inflammation. The beauty industry considers sensitive skin to be that which flushes and blushes easily. It is a delicate skin type that can be a precursor to rosacea. This is why skin care products made for sensitive skin should be soothing and should not contain stimulating ingredients.

Causes of Sensitivity

Dermatologists commonly blame genetics for sensitivity and rosacea. I dislike focusing on genetic factors because it leads people to believe that their sensitivity is unavoidable. While you may have a genetic predisposition to a more stimulated cardiovascular system or a rosacea-prone skin color, you can control inflammation by correcting its cause and balancing your body.

If you have this type of system, including a tendency toward high blood pressure, high pitta, poor digestion, and allergies, you tend to have a stronger blood flow and capillary dilation, which cause breakage and redness. This causes blushing, which may be constant or intermittent and acute, depending on the amount of stimulation. It is also another reason why skin hydration is important, since good water content in its blood and tissues keeps the capillaries flexible and prevents damage. It is a form of protection against easily stimulated blood systems and helps prevent breakouts as well as broken blood vessels.

Along with hydration, skin color can provide protection as well as camouflage for sensitivity. Returning to the point about a predisposition for sensitive skin, your genetic makeup dictates the amount of melanin in your skin, which can make sensitivity more or less visible and provide varying levels of defense against sun exposure. But while higher levels of melanin provides darker skin with more protection from the sun, dark skin is actually more reactive because it has a heightened immune response. This causes hyperpigmentation and inflammation, even though the irritation is less noticeable. Fair complexions appear to have a greater tendency to redness, but this has to do with dehydration and skin thinness, as well as the color itself. Lighter skin has less melanin and therefore a lower immune response to stimuli, which results in less inflammation-induced scarring and pigmentation.

But sensitive skin does not only occur because of a genetic tendency; environmental factors also play an important role in depleting the skin's barrier and making it vulnerable to inflammation. Because sensitivity is accentuated by heat and trauma, external factors such as ultraviolet damage, pollution, wind damage, and temperature fluctuations all contribute to rosacea, eczema, allergic, and sensitive skin.

Sun is probably the most obvious environmental influence on sensitive skin, because sunburn and overexposure to the heat causes direct inflammation and damages cells; it also causes long-term dehydration. In the last chapter, we discussed how sun exposure affects acne-prone skin, and because acne is also a form of inflammation, the same concepts apply here. While the sun's pitta energy promotes sensitivity, many other environmental elements do the same by depleting the skin's resilience. Any form of trauma contributes to sensitivity, and both wind and pollution cause skin damage—wind applying pressure and pollution (including exhaust fumes) wreaking havoc on the cellular level. Extreme temperatures and fluctuations also induce inflammation, because as the skin adjusts to different conditions, the blood vessels dilate and the capillaries sometimes break, leading to chronic redness. This is why some skin becomes more sensitive in the wintertime; the frosty weather outside strongly contrasts with heated indoor conditions. The same goes for the height of summertime when hot outdoor temperatures alternate with cold, air-conditioned rooms. To help make such transitions easier on your skin, pat your face for a few minutes when you move indoors or out and experience different extremes in temperature. This helps regulate skin temperature as you adjust to the new environment.

A number of behaviors also affect sensitive skin. While you may be prone to inflammation, it is usually your lifestyle that sets the stage for chronic redness or skin ailments. Diet is hugely important to managing sensitivities. Alcohol, tobacco, caffeine, spicy foods, fried foods, and overcooked and barbequed foods cause dehydration and capillary dilation, which worsen sensitivity. These pitta-increasing foods create internal heat and aggravate sensitivity, whereas a pitta-pacifying diet soothes and calms redness. Eat lighter foods that do not overwork your digestive system, and opt for cooling, raw foods to reduce skin sensitivity and overall heat, inflammation, and acid in your body. A vegetarian diet is ideal for pittas, but if you do consume animal products, lean meats are best because they are less heavy and require less digestive fire to process them.

Pitta lifestyles and characteristics also promote heat and sensitivity within body tissues. People with rosacea and sensitive skin often put a lot of pressure on themselves and are known perfectionists. These characteristics heighten the heart rate and produce internal heat. According to ayurveda, pitta's tendency to compete, organize, and become agitated also causes stress that stimulates the cardiovascular system. All inflammation is governed by pitta (fire). Pittas put an ample amount of stress on themselves, which overburdens the circulatory system and causes high blood pressure and blood vessel dilation.

Stress also weakens the digestive system. Since the digestive process is governed by pitta, dysfunction in this system can cause excess acid and inflammation. Ayurveda considers undigested food very detrimental to the body, as it is a form of waste. This waste, along with any other factors that tax the body, is the cause of allergic skin. A compromised immune system leads to reactions. Dr. Vasant Lad has said that people who are highly influenced by the weather, have food sensitivities, or suffer from allergic skin reactions demonstrate imbalance; their constitutions cannot cope with any external influence because they are already burdened with toxicity. Emotional distress is just another strain that gives way to inflammation, dehydration, and poor digestion.

Another lifestyle-related influence is a lack of water intake and of adequate hydration in skin care products. Dehydration increases sensitivity because it weakens the skin's acid mantle (barrier function). Think of the skin as a brick wall: The cells (bricks) and the intracellular lipids (mortar) create a dense barrier. When skin cells dehydrate, they shrink, causing tiny spaces or cracks in the wall. This creates weakness, making it easier for bacteria, germs, and other environmental pollutants to infiltrate and for moisture to escape from the deeper cells. Hydration levels can sometimes be linked to genetics, and research shows that Asian skin tends to experience more transepidermal water loss than Caucasian and African-American skin, making it more sensitive. Hyperpigmentation occurs when dehydration allows skin to be irritated constantly and is also a common occurrence in Asian skin.

The use of natural skin care products is important, because they absorb and penetrate better than synthetic products that simply sit on the skin's surface. Hydrating serums and creams are imperative for any skin sensitivity; moisture calms the skin (reduces pitta), and only hydrated skin has the capacity to regenerate and heal itself. Poor skin care can lead to self-induced sensitivity, and overuse or misuse of peels and astringents can lead to cellular damage and a stripping of the skin's natural defenses.

Caring for Sensitive Skin

Proper care is vitally important for sensitive skin. Skin care products should provide protection as well as anti-inflammatory action. When choosing products for sensitive skin, be cautious and avoid any irritating or depleting ingredients that might exacerbate your delicate skin. This may seem obvious, but a lot of sensitivity is self-induced. The use of glycolic peels and a variety of drying agents can weaken the skin and make you photosensitive. If your skin has visible redness, avoid chemical peels and other products with drying agents and opt for a gentle exfoliant, such as a scrub made of soft jojoba beads and a clay spot treatment for actual pustules.

Using natural, gentle skin care products geared toward calming and soothing is another component of daily maintenance for sensitive skin. Petroleum-based products are clogging (comedogenic), which suffocates the skin and prevents it from being healthy and resilient. Petrolatum and propylene glycol are also common irritants; many people think they "react to everything," when they actually just need to use products without petrochemicals. Synthetic fragrances and dyes can also inflame or deplete the skin; I have seen localized inflammation on eyelids and cheeks where color cosmetics have been applied and near earlobes where perfumes have been dabbed. A pure mineral makeup line is the best alternative when selecting eye shadows and blushes, and natural perfumes made of high-quality essential oils are ideal. The latter is especially important because studies have found that some perfumes increase photosensitivity.

However, you must be careful even when using natural ingredients. Stimulating herbs and additives such as ginseng, vitamin C, and lemon essential oil cause redness in sensitive skin. Try to incorporate as many natural, comforting ingredients as possible. Essential oil of sandalwood, chamomile, helichryse, calendula, melissa, and lavender all lessen inflammation. Nourishing base oils such as jojoba, evening primrose, coconut, and borage bolster the skin's immunity to damage and offer a lubricating barrier. Vitamin E oil is another excellent ingredient for healing after trauma; it is an antioxidant, which helps strengthen the skin.

From a more scientific standpoint, collagen and elastin in skin care products are fantastic additions for rebuilding skin tissue. Collagen increases the water content of the skin, which also makes it more healthy. But finding and using products with a natural base is still imperative; without this, they will not be able to properly permeate the skin surface.

Rosacea

Rosacea is an extreme form of sensitivity that is actually a cardiovascular disorder, appearing as red skin, sometimes with papules and a thickened texture. It always presents with dilated or broken capillaries, and because the blood nourishes and detoxifies the skin, the dysfunction of blood vessels causes the other rosacea symptoms of skin nodules and deformation (in severe cases). Rosacea leads to couperose, a condition in which dilated blood vessels retain blood cells, giving an appearance of redness; this is caused by poor elasticity of the capillary walls. All rosacea, sensitivity, and broken capillaries include couperose. Rosacea is becoming more common as more people are exposed to extreme weather and lifestyle stress.

Rosacea (known as "acne rosacea") has four identified degrees of severity. Some rosacea manifests as subtle flushing. This is an early stage, and if you do not care for your skin and pacify your pitta at this point, it will progress to a more intensive form of the ailment. Stage one is referred to as prerosacea, when the skin exhibits signs of sensitivity, with occasional blushing and flushing. You can prevent the condition from worsening at this point if you avoid external triggers, use proper skin care, and mitigate internal inflammation.

Stage two is mild rosacea. The skin becomes highly sensitive and prone to flushing with heated inflammation. Irritation in this stage lasts for several hours but is not permanent.

Stage three, moderate rosacea, is when redness becomes chronic. The skin is easily aggravated, with stinging, burning inflammation. Acnelike bumps that do not come to a head and are full of lymphatic fluid may appear chronically or flare up during times of stress or in extreme weather; broken blood vessels are apparent.

This leads to stage four, severe rosacea. Luckily, only a minority of sufferers progress to this stage, when papules and tissue deformation occur. Bulbous noses are usually found in men, often induced by constant, excessive alcohol consumption (which is an identified rosacea trigger as well as a pitta aggravator).

CAUSES OF ROSACEA

As mentioned earlier, ayurveda believes that rosacea is always related to the cardiovascular system and is the result of a pitta imbalance. This is why both Eastern and Western physicians agree that rosacea sufferers (like those with sensitive skin) should avoid things that stimulate the heart rate. This includes eating spicy and barbecued foods, drinking alcoholic beverages, smoking, doing excessive cardiovascular workouts, exposing themselves to extreme heat or cold (which dilates the capillaries), and subjecting themselves to constant stress. These behaviors not only contribute to the aggravation and advancement of rosacea due to the accumulation of heat in the body, but they can also lead to acute rosacea breakouts.

Poor digestion and elimination also contribute to rosacea, since pitta governs digestion. Ensuring that you are properly digesting your food and purging waste greatly improves this condition. The first time one of my clients broke out in papulopustular rosacea (rosacea with papules), she was so determined to heal her skin that she started a series of colon irrigation treatments and completely eliminated allergens and difficult-to-digest foods from her life. The results were incredible. After approximately one year, I couldn't even tell she had had rosacea! Though it was a struggle, with patience and natural treatments, she attained beautiful, healthy skin without oral medication or topical prescriptions.

CONVENTIONAL TREATMENTS FOR ROSACEA

While rosacea varies in degree of severity from person to person, dermatologists tend to treat all cases in the same way. Oral antibiotics, like tetracycline, and topical antibiotics, such as metronidazole (found under the brand name Metrogel), are commonly prescribed to relieve symptoms. But these solutions are temporary if not counterproductive. Metronidazole can damage skin and even worsen rosacea. According to ayurveda, antibiotics aggravate pitta, which is the original cause of rosacea. Although they are prescribed for their anti-inflammatory properties, common side effects such as photosensitivity, heartburn, diarrhea, nausea, and liver toxicity (all symptoms of pitta excess) indicate that any reduction in inflammation is short-lived.

When treating the skin tissue itself, lasers and intense pulsed light (IPL) therapy are also popular recommendations, and they can be used to eliminate damaged capillaries. But this is purely cosmetic, and these treatments do not prevent or cure the root cause of the problem. Redness and broken blood vessels simply return if the underlying inflammatory issues are not resolved. Laser and IPL treatments are best practiced in conjunction with a program of internal healing to produce long-term results.

HOLISTIC SOLUTIONS FOR ROSACEA

According to ayurveda, most skin disorders, especially rosacea, are linked to dysfunction of the rakta dhatu (blood, specifically the red blood cells). The blood is governed by pitta, and the reduction of internal heat pacifies this dosha and puts less stress on the blood vessels in the face.

One of the best ways to relieve rosacea is to change the way you eat. Everything you ingest influences the energetic components of your body, so following a pitta-pacifying diet is imperative. Many of my rosacea clients have felt it was nearly impossible to give up coffee, wine, or chocolate, but until these stimulants were eliminated, they saw little improvement in their skin. (See the food chart on p. 41) Avoiding hot, spicy foods and acidic fruits and vegetables is the first step, but you must also consider how your food is prepared. Because oil enhances heat, reducing pitta also means using oil sparingly when cooking. Many pittas cannot digest fats properly, and too much oil consumption aggravates the liver. Also, avoid adding heat to your food through overcooking, frying, and barbequing. These cooking methods not only increase the presence of the fire dosha in your meal, but they often make the food difficult to digest. When you overwork your digestive system, it requires more digestive fire and creates heat. Al dente or raw vegetables and gently cooked proteins are ideal. You also need to be strict about avoiding any foods to which you have allergies or sensitivities, since the energy required to process them also causes inflammation.

Because rosacea is a cardiovascular disorder, you must address imbalances within this system. The appearance of broken and dilated capillaries shows that your circulatory system is distressed, very likely congested, and in need of detoxification. Blood-cleansing herbs such as turmeric, arjuna, hibiscus, coriander (cilantro), burdock root, neem, and amalaki are excellent. Each of these remedies is known to purify the blood and relieve it of pitta heat. If you have trouble finding them at health food stores or specialty herb shops, try one of the many online retailers that sell ayurvedic staples (see the resources section at the back of this book). The herbs can be taken in capsule or powder form, but they can also be gently introduced into your everyday routine as teas or cold infusions. Tinctures are sometimes an option, but most tinctures have an alcohol base, and alcohol aggravates pitta.

Two of my favorite remedies are hibiscus tea and a coriander cold infusion; both are easy to make and delicious. Hibiscus is relatively easy to find in tea bags, but I buy dry hibiscus flowers from tea specialty stores or herb shops. I simply steep a heaping tablespoonful in boiling water for five to ten minutes, resulting in a slightly tart tea with a lovely, rich red color. I strain it before drinking; I also sometimes chill it to make a wonderful iced tea in summertime. Hibiscus is an excellent anti-inflammatory and also lowers high blood pressure.

A coriander cold infusion is just as straightforward to prepare, but it is more of an acquired taste because of its unique flavor. To make this cooling drink, place approximately two tablespoons of chopped fresh coriander leaves in a glass of water and let it sit overnight. In the morning, remove the leaves, and strain the coriander-laced liquid. According to ayurveda, this pitta-pacifying beverage decreases heat in the blood and purifies the body of heavy metals. It can also be used on a compress for inflamed skin.

Blood cleansing can also by done by bloodletting. This is an excellent treatment for relieving the body of blood laden with heat and can be done by placing suction devices on the surface of the skin or by donating blood. Both ayurveda and traditional Chinese medicine (TCM) use suction for bloodletting; ayurveda employs animal horns or leeches, and TCM uses glass cups. Practitioners commonly place these items on areas of the back, and the areas that become reddest indicate the body parts and organs that store the most heat and toxicity. Not only does this practice release excess pitta in the affected organs, but it also shows where the weakest points of the body are, which can help you choose more specific cleanses or rejuvenating therapies geared toward those organs. When all of the covered areas are very red, it indicates that the blood is saddled with heat that must be alleviated.

One way to do this is through pranayama (breath work). This helps bring more oxygen to the blood and purge heat via exhalation. These breathing exercises are both purifying and cooling, and pranayama is incredibly good for stress reduction, which is another big trigger of rosacea and sensitive skin. Simple exercises can slow down the heart rate and increase oxygen intake. Try inhaling for a count of ten, hold the breath for another count of ten, then exhale slowly to a last count of ten. I used to do this ten times every night before bed when I had acne and found that it helped me sleep better and decreased inflammation.

One client and yogini I know does *sheetali pranayama* when she is feeling hot-headed or irritable. This is a traditional breathing exercise specifically aimed at ridding the body of excess heat by rolling the sides of the tongue up, making a cooling tunnel through which breath can enter the body. I have done this breathing exercise when I've had acid stomach and when I've felt irritable. It doesn't make a lot of noise, so you can do it anywhere. Sit comfortably and roll your tongue to make a tube. This acts like a straw through which you breathe. Inhale through your mouth, allowing the air to travel through your rolled tongue, picking up coolness along the way. Exhale through your nose. Feel the cold breath coming into your body and excess heat leaving it.

Finally, beyond keeping your mind and body cool, you need to address the lymphatic system. While heat may be concentrated in the circulatory system and too much stimulation here is detrimental to rosacea, lymphatic congestion and water retention also contribute to the dilation and breakage of capillaries.

Overweight people sometimes have a lot of inflammation on the cheeks, possibly due to superficial dehydration caused by a lack of circulation. Here, blood is not moving freely through the capillaries, and the lymph is not draining. When people with kapha imbalances (but not necessarily kapha constitutions) who are prone to congestion and puffiness swell with lymphatic fluid, pressure is put on the blood vessels, dilating and breaking them. This is prevalent in the thigh area, creating spider veins, and in other areas where cellulite exists, further inhibiting circulation. When lymphatic congestion cuts off circulation, dehydration and undernourished skin cells result. This exacerbates inflammation and worsens rosacea. When blood vessels break, this too compromises proper circulation in the skin. While blood flow is supposed to nourish skin tissue and transport waste away from it, poor circulation impedes the skin's ability to self-cleanse and detoxify. This gives way to the formation of nodules and skin bumps; it also further inhibits lymphatic movement.

Lymphatic drainage is important for sustaining a healthy complexion and soothing sensitive skin. Pressure-point massage often drains off lymphatic and glandular congestion almost immediately, bringing down redness. To do this on your own, simply press and release sections of your skin with all four fingertips on both hands. Start at the top of your forehead, forming pressure-point rows with your fingers, and work your way down until you reach the underside of your chin. Pay special attention to the "rows" on the brow bone and under the cheekbones. Avoid going over your eyes, as this area is tender, but spend time on the bones of the eye socket, as this can help relieve puffiness around the eyes.

Skin Care for Rosacea

When it comes to rosacea, hydration is the first line of defense, so it is imperative to avoid astringent skin care products. Use a milk cleanser to avoid disturbing the skin's acid mantle, and only use hydrating, alcohol-free toners. Hydrating serums are also essential; choose one containing soothing ingredients such as aloe vera or chamomile water. Rosewater is particularly beneficial for rosacea, because it helps repair and strengthen capillary walls; make sure it is high quality and completely pure, because some cheaper, low-quality rosewaters are extracted with chemical solvents that can actually be irritating.

The more water you can infuse into your skin, the healthier, more robust, and less easily aggravated it will become. The more dehydrated your skin, the easier it is for blood vessels to break. Use nonstimulating oils (such as coconut and jojoba) and soothing balms to help keep your capillaries supple and barricade moisture in.

Rosacea skin that is severely dehydrated has a tendency to become so sensitive that it cannot tolerate oils and creams. Skin like this usually feels tight and is rough to the touch, and even anti-inflammatory oils cause skin reactions and burning sensations. This occurs because dehydration compromises the skin's barrier, and the fats in the oils have heating qualities that penetrate deeply. Even oils that are good for pitta can be aggravating, so if you think your skin is dehydrated, test a little oil on one patch of skin before applying it all over your face. If you can't use oil, opt for a lotion to replenish your skin, and incorporate heavier moisturizers when the rosacea has begun to calm down and your skin has healed.

Sunblock is extremely important for rosacea skin, which is aggravated by UV damage. Limit sun exposure even when you apply sunblock because the thermal heat itself inflames rosacea. Use a natural, mineral-based sunblock; many chemical sunscreen agents are irritating.

Conventional medicine often stresses that people with rosacea must only use noncomedogenic skin care (products that will not clog pores). If you use products made wholly of natural ingredients, this should never be a problem. Rosacea skin is prone to dehydration because excess pitta burns up moisture. This leads to dried sebum in the skin. Again, it is important to remember that it isn't oil, but a lack of water, that causes congestion. Try increasing the moisture of your skin with water-rich serums, and get regular facial treatments that include carefully performed extractions. Extractions should be followed by a soothing, nurturing mask treatment.

Use a calming mask once or twice a week at home to cool the skin and boost hydration. Gel masks are packed with water and a good option for rosacea; you might also try cream masks that contain pitta-pacifying oils. Cream masks have more body and are ideal during the colder, drier months. If you do not have a cream mask in your skin care collection, yogurt is a great homemade treatment for rosacea and sensitive skin. It reduces pitta whether you eat it or use it topically. Simply apply a tablespoon of plain, organic yogurt to the skin and leave it on for thirty minutes. Rinse with cool to tepid water, and pat dry with gentle pressing motions. Your skin should feel more moist and calmer. This is an excellent mask for rashes and irritated breakouts.

As with generally sensitive skin, the holistic approach for rosacea must encompass a soothing skin care regimen, along with anti-inflammatory lifestyle practices such as stress management, a cooling (pitta-reducing) diet, and avoidance of stimulants (including tobacco, alcohol, and caffeine). Since both rosacea and sensitive skin have multiple causes, this approach appropriately addresses the body, mind, and spirit.

Eczema

Eczema is very common, but it is often undiagnosed because many people mistake it for an allergic reaction. This skin ailment can exhibit different symptoms, depending on the type of eczema you have and what you use on your skin. It can show up as dry, flaky patches of skin; red lesions that are inflamed and accompanied by a burning sensation; or small bumps that look like water blisters and may be itchy. Eczema is often so irritating that it wakes you up during the night. Changes of season can trigger it, as can food allergies and skin care products, but these are not the root causes. Eczema, like other skin ailments, is an expression of doshic imbalance. The solution is not simply to eliminate the symptoms but to discover what is happening inside the body.

Eczema Triggers

According to modern dermatology, there is no official cause for eczema. While cortisone creams are usually the prescribed solution for eczema outbreaks, avoiding triggers often proves more effective.

Extreme dehydration has been the trigger for every case of eczema I have observed. When the skin is dried out, it is vulnerable to irritants and bacteria (leading to eczema bumps). When the internal organs are dehydrated, many imbalances result, causing inflammation, a backup of waste, and tissue depletion.

Skin that is prone to eczema flares up when its defenses are compromised, and depending on the type of eczema, aggravated doshas may manifest as dryness, redness, or dampness. This is why air travel, which leads to excess vata and dehydration, often triggers eczema. The combination of experiencing a new climate, the dry airplane environment, and the stress of traveling provide a perfect formula for a flare-up. If you are prone to eczema, lubricate your skin when taking a long flight and spray it frequently with a hydrosol plant water to avoid breakouts. This is even beneficial if you do not have eczema, because constant flying and traveling ages the skin rapidly.

Stress management is important in avoiding dehydration and other eczema triggers. As we discussed earlier, stress weakens the kidneys and leads to internal inflammation that can translate into topical inflammation (in the form of pitta eczema, which is red and irritated). Stress-related eczema often occurs on the insides of the elbows, between the fingers, and on the backs of the knees. Posttraumatic stress disorder has also been cited as an eczema trigger, demonstrating how closely this skin disorder is linked to emotional states.

Eczema breakouts are most likely to occur during a change of season or climate when the body is stressed by the need to reacclimatize. Kapha blisters usually appear during shifts from dry to wet environments. Vata eczema occurs when going from hot to cold, dry weather. But again, climate change is only a trigger, because the external environment causes any doshic imbalance to show up as symptoms. Furthermore, the qualities of these symptoms reflect the qualities of the imbalance.

TYPES OF ECZEMA AND THEIR AYURVEDIC SOLUTIONS

The conventional protocol for managing eczema uses cortisone cream to reduce redness. Unfortunately, this thins the skin without treating the source of the imbalance. Treating the appropriate doshas is more effective than cookie-cutter prescriptions, and because there are different types of eczema (corresponding to vata, pitta, and kapha), understanding them helps you identify the best way to treat whichever form you have.

Skin with vata eczema is dry, flaky, and chapped, but it is also the easiest type to treat. While it can appear on the face, behind the ears, and in other small areas on the body, it often occurs in parts that have been depleted by wind exposure and other elemental damage. Large areas such as the sides of the midriff, the calves, and the lower arms and hands can display this type of eczema. Vata eczema does not itch or burn, but it can become uncomfortable if the skin becomes so dry that it starts to crack.

Apply a rich cream or pure oil for this condition; it helps immensely and feels wonderful. Ensure that you use only pure vegetable oils so your skin can absorb them fully. Sesame, sunflower, and avocado oils are especially effective because of their heavy texture, and moisturizing this type of eczema is like a refreshing drink for the skin.

Internal moisturizing is also important, and I recommend taking omega-3 essential fatty acids. They are fantastic for lubricating the intestines, holding hydration, and aiding digestion. Remember, oil is not water-soluble, so it will help retain water.

Pitta eczema is red and inflamed, and sufferers often experience a burning sensation. It most often appears on the face and hands, but it can also spread to other areas of the body. Although it can be dry and flaky with obvious skin irritation, you must avoid straight oils and rich creams when experiencing a breakout (unlike with vata eczema). Oil accentuates pitta's heat and creates hivelike lesions. Think of frying food—you use oil to make the pan hotter. Even cooling oils seem to aggravate pitta inflammation. Instead, try a gel moisturizer containing aloe vera and a light lotion. You may need to reapply it throughout the day to keep your skin moist and support its barrier function. Spraying hydrosols of rose and chamomile can also be very effective.

My own desperation in dealing with an eczema outbreak led to the discovery of Pure + simple's best-selling pitta eczema product. Excess pitta had brought years of acne as well as eczema. In treating eczema outbreaks, I had used emollients that only increased heat and caused hivelike reactions. During one flare-up, I hastily applied Pure + simple Firming Eye Gel—and it was fantastic! Because it is nourishing to combat aging and light in texture so it can be used in the sensitive eye area, it provided protection and moisture without heat-inducing oil. After this product was reintroduced as our Skin Softening Moisture Lotion, it became our most popular moisturizer for sensitive skin.

Skin care products that contain algae are also beneficial for pitta eczema. The algae holds in moisture without the need for a heavy cream or oil. Many serums and moisturizers contain algae for this reason; simply look for it in the ingredients list when shopping for skin care products. The closer it is to the top of the list, the more algae the product contains.

After the appearance of pitta eczema subsides, you can use oils and richer moisturizers again; this is actually advisable because preventing dehydration with oil-based skin care helps prevent the occurrence of pitta eczema breakouts.

Ingesting and cooking with cooling oils, especially organic coconut oil, is ideal for pitta eczema. Take or use one to two tablespoons of oil a day to give your body more moisture and provide anti-inflammatory and antibacterial properties. This type of eczema requires you to pacify pitta, so you need to eat and manage your emotions according to pitta- reducing guidelines. One helpful practice is to avoid alcohol in your skin care products as well as in your diet. Because alcohol adds heat and dehydrates, it is extremely aggravating to this type of eczema.

Kapha eczema looks wet, like light perspiration on the skin, and is at high risk for fungal infection. Usually it acquires what appear to be water blisters and is very itchy. Keep this type of eczema clean and use antibacterial, antifungal, purifying herbs such as tea tree, peppermint, and sage in the form of hydrosols or diluted in oil or lotion. These herbs can also be found in many natural skin care products aimed at purifying the skin.

As with any antikapha skin care regimen, you need to avoid kapha qualities in products. This means avoiding all rich, moist skin care. Never apply heavy creams and oils to this type of eczema, especially when water-filled bumps appear. Dusting turmeric powder on the affected area can help absorb some of the skin's wetness and also kills localized bacteria. Products containing black mud and dead sea minerals, which contain sulfur, are also excellent for kapha eczema because of their antimicrobial properties. One popular Pure + simple moisturizer contains black mud and can be used on eczema on the face, hands, and back of the ears. Clients have called it "amazing" and "a lifesaver," but not all dead sea products are created equal. Some companies use a petroleum-derived chemical base, which is counterproductive and results in clogged pores. Remember to avoid any skin care products that contain petrolatum, mineral oil, or the words *propyl* or *paraffinium* in the ingredients list.

Consuming flax seed oil is excellent for this type of eczema; it mitigates kapha and lowers cholesterol and fat in the body. Take one or two tablespoons (or the equivalent in capsules) each day to help clear up outbreaks and prevent future ones. Avoid fermented foods such as alcohols, preserves, vinegars, and miso, which aggravate kapha and internal fungus (candida). Kapha eczema is provoked by dampness, fungus, yeast, and mold—all of which you must avoid and eliminate from your body and environment. One of my clients broke out in kapha eczema after moving into a basement apartment that had a mold problem. The dampness of the basement and the presence of mold resulted in a topical reaction expressing excess kapha. When she moved again, her skin cleared up quickly.

Eczema is sometimes difficult to diagnose because it can come and go. Just remember that when you experience a breakout of vata, pitta, or kapha eczema, there is a doshic imbalance at work. Adapting how you care for your skin and body in accordance with which dosha(s) need balance is the only way to truly treat eczema. This approach also helps clear up your skin over the long term and avoid cyclical, recurring eczema.

Eight

Aging Skin

We are always aging. Many people fear growing older because they do not understand that *aging* is simply *changing*. Stopping this process is a futile goal and stifles personal growth. Aging is just a reminder that the body is a vessel, something we cannot fully control. As we move closer to wisdom, we move away from the physical. Our mind expands with life experience, while our body degenerates, mirroring a balance that exists in everything.

Nevertheless, modern-day demands and expectations also govern us. Our youth-obsessed society motivates us to be combative against aging, but we must revise our goal of antiaging to one of rejuvenation—supporting the process of maturation and promoting healthy tissue. For best results, we must treat our skin topically and revitalize ourselves from the inside with both physical and emotional rejuvenation measures.

What Is Aging?

When it comes to skin aging, most people generally identify a list of symptoms that simply indicate that their bodies have been lived in. Inflammation accumulates from a lifetime of energy expended and shows up as fine lines and damaged texture. Long-term exposure to the elements causes broken capillaries and "age spots." And the slowing down of internal systems results in less circulation and reduced collagen, elastin, and sebum production, all of which result in dull, dehydrated, weakened skin. Signs of aging are external markers of an internal shift. Wrinkles, jowls, and loss of skin tone indicate that we have stopped developing and have entered the age of experience.

It is natural for tissues to sag and internal systems to become exhausted with living, but if you take care of your body, mind, and spirit, you can evolve gracefully. To age in the healthiest way possible, you must look at the aging process and its most important factors. Then you can understand how to support your body's tissues and the logic behind popular antiaging methods. The two facets we will focus on are slowed metabolism and inflammation.

With age, the body slows down. While a twenty-five-year-old's skin cell turnover occurs approximately every twenty-eight days, a seventy-five-year-old's occurs about every ninety days. This means the skin does not renew as often and causes an accumulation of dead skin cells on the surface, which promotes dryness. The skin and body look less youthful with this decrease in cellular renewal, which is why exfoliation is used so often in antiaging products and services.

But it is not only cell turnover that slows; the healing process does too. After age twenty-five, there is a drastic drop in collagen and elastin production. Collagen dictates the hydration and thickness of the skin, while elastin governs firmness and elasticity; their decline results in a loss of moisture, tissue, and tone.

As we mature, our silhouette changes, and body fat increases as muscle tone and bone mass decrease. This is because metabolism and ossification have slowed down. Not only does this affect how our body looks, but it also contributes to more skin sagging. With a decrease in muscle and bone mass, the structure under the skin becomes smaller, creating what the beauty industry calls "redundant skin." No amount or type of antiaging skin care can remedy this situation.

As all the body's systems slow down, detoxification and waste removal become less rapid, and blockages accumulate. These blockages manifest as skin deposits, chronic constipation, or (in ayurvedic philosophy) a stagnation of energy in the energetic pathways. According to ayurveda, we all have nonphysical, energetic passages that allow energy to be dispersed throughout our bodies. Marma points are the junctions where the mind, body, and energy meet on our bodies. When our energy becomes obstructed, circulation is impeded; the skin receives less nourishment; and the body gets colder, especially the hands and feet. Exercise helps prevent the stagnation that hampers energy and blood flow, but it's important to note that slower forms of exercise such as yoga, tai chi, and qi gong are just as effective (if not more so) as intensive, fast-paced workouts.

Certain types of alternative therapies also keep circulation and energy moving, so they are fantastic as antiaging measures. Ayurveda uses a technique called *marmani* (or simply, *marma*), in which specific points on the body are massaged to stimulate corresponding internal organs, doshas, and energies. I have used this therapy when performing facials; pressing certain marma points on the face can reduce puffiness and drain lymphatic fluid. Acupuncture is similar to marmani, as it serves to break up stagnation and open the energetic pathways. Acupuncture facials are a recent trend in antiaging beauty care, and the results are excellent; as with marmani, the focus is on dispersing blockages and increasing stimulation.

The other cause of aging is inflammation, an inevitable response to crisis or damage. Sun exposure, trauma, and stress inflame the body and tissues, resulting in deterioration in the joints, muscles, and skin. Inflammation creates free radicals—molecules that damage skin tissue—and also stresses and breaks the capillaries. Not only do broken capillaries create redness and unsightly damaged vessels, but they compromise the circulation. Inflammation also puts pressure on the skin, producing fine lines and wrinkles.

Diet is a factor in creating heat and inflammation. Meat is acidic and hard to digest, inflaming the internal organs. Refined sugar has the same effect, leading experts such as the renowned dermatologist and author Dr. Nicholas Perricone to conclude in his book *The Perricone Prescription* that it causes wrinkles. Christina Pirello, a nutritionist, whole-food advocate, and author, agrees with this link between excess glucose consumption and aging. In her book *Glow*, she writes that age spots are another result of too much sugar; they form when the body tries to expel simple carbohydrates. Because of this overload, fat blocks melanin, dispersing pigment in an uneven pattern.

The endocrine system is another factor, and many women experience inflammation because of hormonal changes that cause an imbalance. This is especially true during perimenopause. Once menopause occurs, the imbalance tends to right itself but the metabolic slowdown becomes accentuated.

Menopause

Menopause causes drastic changes in women's bodies as they pass from the child-bearing stage into the more reflective years. Many women see this change as depressing, because it becomes increasingly difficult to maintain youthful-looking skin as estrogen levels drop and tone and suppleness decrease. The absence of estrogen also lets testosterone flourish, causing excess hair growth on the upper lip and chin. Instead of viewing this change as a loss of beauty, we should celebrate it as a transition. It marks the end of child-bearing years, which are so often associated with femininity, sexuality, and desirability (in women), but beauty extends beyond this two-dimensional definition. To deny this is harmful and self-defeating, because all women inevitably experience this shift as they mature. When we view beauty as good health and strive for this instead of attempting to hang on to youth, we promote a more loving, self-accepting perception of attractiveness.

According to ayurveda, the transition into menopause is a vata time. It is a change from one phase to another, and vata governs the energy of change and movement. This means many women may experience characteristics of vata dysfunction: scattered mental patterns, forget-fulness, oversensitivity to their surroundings, and insomnia. Vata phys-ical aspects can increase; the skin and hair may become thinner, more coarse, duller, and drier, while the bones become more brittle. But it is also during this transition that other dosha imbalances become more obvious. Women with high pitta experience hot flashes, breakouts, and moodiness, while those with kapha accumulation experience wa-ter retention and lethargy.

As we approach menopause, we need to calm our vata dosha and support this beautiful time of transformation. This approach is good for antiaging in general, because the vata we accumulate as we age causes overall tissue depletion.

With the dramatic decrease in estrogen, osteoporosis becomes a concern, because estrogen facilitates the bones' absorption of calcium from the blood and inhibits its loss. According to ayurveda, osteoporo-sis is caused by high vata, along with an increase in *asthi agni* (the "fire," or metabolic energy, that governs bone tissue), as the body tries to compensate for reduced estrogen. Shatavari is an excellent herb for in-creasing and mimicking natural estrogen, and it also pacifies vata. This ayurvedic supplement is a staple for supporting the female reproduc-tive system, and it can be taken as a tea, in capsules, or by the spoonful (powdered). The standard dose is two tablespoons twice a day (or the equivalent in capsule form), but you should consult an ayurvedic practitioner beforehand to ensure that this is the right remedy for you. Be careful when addressing and treating your endocrine system, whether you are taking herbal or pharmaceutical medications.

Topical skin care plays a huge role in making an effortless transition into menopause, and massaging your body with sesame oil every day is best for pacifying vata. Pay special attention to your scalp as it also calms your nervous system when applied here. Apply an oil-rich moisturizer to your face to protect the skin and compensate for lower sebum production. A pure face oil containing evening primrose is especially good for menopause.

Support this oiling by pairing it with increased hydration to further reduce vata symptoms. Using a serum containing hyaluronic acid helps make up for a decrease in estrogen and diminishes fine lines and dryness, as do relaxing practices such as spending time in a steam room or wet sauna. Total body steaming moistens vata, lubricates the tissues, and calms the mind.

But topical care alone is not enough for adequate hydration. Protecting the kidneys is critical. The kidneys influence water metabolism and dispersion as well as growth, development, and reproduction. The latter makes them very important during menopause (when kidney energy is exhausted). They are governed by vata and are vulnerable during this time, so you need to support and nurture them by monitoring your water intake, keeping your lower and middle back warm, and avoiding excess salt.

The right diet can also pacify vata, and eating moist, grounding foods is important for absorbing and retaining water in the body, skin, and cells. Watery stews and hearty vegetables help keep the gastrointestinal tract moist. Foods with estrogenic properties—including spices like turmeric, oregano, and thyme, as well as whole-grain cereals, soy, and flaxseed—are also helpful.

Resting both your mind and body is imperative when trying to balance vata during and after menopause. Rest itself supports any transition, so try to go to bed early, but be careful not to oversleep or sleep during the day, since this causes a kapha imbalance. Meditation is another powerful tool in grounding your energy and focus; it spurs self-reflection and can help you welcome this life change.

Effects of Aging

Now that we have discussed what causes the signs of aging, we should also talk about how this directly affects tissues and skin cells.

Decreased Collagen, Fine Lines, and Dehydration

When the subject of antiaging comes up, collagen is always mentioned. This protein makes up 70 percent of the dermis layer of the skin and the fibers of other connective tissues. It is composed of three chains of twisted polypeptides, each of which contains approximately one hundred amino acid units arranged in a defined sequence.

The drastic drop in collagen production in a woman's midtwenties is just another indication of slowing metabolism. With age, collagen also loses its suppleness and its cross-links with other collagen strands, becoming rigid as the structures harden. With the onset of this rigidity, the skin loses its pliability.

But maturation is not the only factor that causes collagen to break down. Estrogen makes cells more vulnerable to inflammation, so birth control pills and other hormonal medications play a role in collagen's production and quality. Too much estrogen can result in thinning skin and contributes to water retention (which may lead to cellulite).

Conversely, the right amount of estrogen improves the skin's texture, making it smoother, moister, and firmer due to an increase in hyaluronic acid. It is hyaluronic acid that strengthens the skin's resistance to stretching and increases its softness and resilience. Many skin care companies are exploring the effectiveness and safety of using estrogen in antiaging skin care for postmenopausal women.

SLACK ELASTIN

Elastin is the protein responsible for skin's elasticity, and it makes up 5 percent of the dermis layer. A lack of elastin causes loss of tone and promotes stretch marks. Elastin is a lighter molecule than collagen, which it supports, and has a weblike structure that weaves in and out, binding collagen strands together. Therefore, the health of elastin determines the skin's firmness.

As we mature, elastin calcifies and loses its flexibility. Sagging or loose skin is caused by elastase (an agent that breaks down elastin). Inflammation stimulates elastase production, demonstrating another way that inflammation causes skin damage and aging.

Some dietary additions can help support elastin; beans and soy are elastase inhibitors, making them excellent antiaging foods. Soy oil is an especially beneficial additive to any skin care formulation.

FREE RADICAL DAMAGE

Free radicals are atoms or molecules with one or more unpaired electron. Because oxygen has two unpaired electrons, it reacts with free radicals. While most oxygen in the body is broken down and used to produce energy, the little that is left over causes chaos in the body.

Free radicals are a major factor in aging, damaging cell membranes, phospholipids, proteins, and DNA and causing pigmented lesions. They also create what is referred to as "smoker's skin" by breaking down fatty acids and forming lipofuscin, which gives the skin a yellow hue. Free radicals are produced by pollution, smoking, stress, adrenal breakdown, exposure to ultraviolet light, and skin irritation. Essentially, they are a product of inflammation.

There are several types of free radicals. One common free radical is called superoxide. Superoxide is formed by UV radiation, some enzyme reactions, inflammation, and sunburn. It is known to attack enzymes and cell membranes, causing them to break down. A cell's membrane governs what passes in and out, and superoxide alters this function, weakening the cell's protection. This weakening allows disease and free radicals to permeate our cells causing signs of skin aging. These signs of aging, such as fine lines, wrinkles, and rough texture, are a result of tissue damage from oxidative stress and attacks to our cells' DNA. Superoxide is also the free radical most responsible for lipofuscin.

With free radicals attacking us, the role of antioxidants is crucial. Vitamin E is one that quenches and neutralizes hydroxyl radicals, and vitamin C regenerates vitamin E that has been destroyed by free radicals. Vitamin C is also instrumental in the creation of superoxide dismutase, an enzyme and antioxidant that lessens the damage of superoxide by converting it into hydrogen peroxide and oxygen; it repairs damaged cells and acts as an anti-inflammatory.

Singlet oxygen is another common free radical. It is produced when oxygen has elevated energy due to absorption of ultraviolet or even fluorescent light. When exposed to UV rays, the skin must deal with singlet oxygen. While the body usually overcomes this attack, when its antioxidant defense is overwhelmed, tissue damage results. Vitamin E, uric acid, beta-carotene, and ubiquinone all fight singlet oxygen by quenching it. When this free radical is quenched it protects our skin from its injury, preventing wrinkles and sun damage.

Conventional Antiaging Solutions and Treatments

Any antiaging solution must include goals. Goals provide expectations as well as limitations and boundaries. A plan can be as simple as tailoring your at-home skin care to your individual needs, or you may desire the results of more extreme treatments. Your plan of action must outline how much energy, effort, and money you intend to invest. Naturally, better results often require a greater investment. Extreme treatments may also be more painful, requiring proper preparation and posttherapy care.

Remember that skin care should be practiced with a view to the overall health of your body and mind. Because health is beauty, nurturing yourself is an antiaging practice. The choice between an intense treatment protocol or a simple regimen depends on your personal values and goals.

Because of our society's demand, antiaging technology is advancing so rapidly that professionals can hardly keep up. The industry's search for youthful skin is so far-reaching that some technology such as laser and IPL therapy has even been derived from military research. The following are popular treatments that are currently available.

Botulinum Toxin (Botox)

Botox has made a splash in the last five years due to its fantastic results. Injections atrophy the facial muscles, preventing them from contracting to make wrinkling movements. This makes your face look more relaxed and facial lines less pronounced. Results of this treatment are temporary, and the injections must be done every few months to maintain results.

But despite its popularity, Botox is derived from botulinum toxin A, a poisonous bacterium that can cause death in large doses. In fact, botulinum toxin A is arguably one of the most toxic substances in existence, and the FDA has issued a warning on the use of cosmetic botox after fatalities of children using the injectable because muscle spasms occured. Beyond this, a study conducted by the University of Calgary found that botox injections do not stay isolated to the targeted area. Instead the botox spreads to surrounding areas and causes atrophy in nontarget muscles. This highlights the risk of habitual botox use, as it can cause loss of control over facial muscles.

Botox is really just a superficial cover-up of an underlying problem, and paralyzing your facial muscles to temporarily stop producing wrinkles is not a good solution. Some women in their twenties and thirties are even getting preventive Botox injections. Not only is this detrimental to their health, but it reflects how willing they are to risk their well-being in the pursuit of "beauty."

FILLERS

Injected fillers are another way to treat wrinkles by, as the name implies, "filling" them in. The injectable sector of the beauty industry is always being updated, so you should do a lot of research before choosing this option. While some fillers come from human tissue, others that claim to be natural come from cows (bovine collagen) and birds (avian collagen). You must assess these ingredients before permitting them to be used on your face or body.

Topical side effects can include allergic reaction, the appearance of lumps and clumps of collagen, infection, and rejection of the filler by the immune system. Some of my clients have had Restylane injections in their lips that resulted in hard, uneven lumps under the skin. This, of course, is counterproductive. Fillers are temporary and, like Botox, must be injected regularly to maintain results.

SURGERY

Face lifts and other cosmetic enhancements are a more extreme option, but not one that I disregard. While these procedures traumatize the skin, the decision to undergo them comes back to your own expectations and goals. Even some of our more "natural-focused" clients at Pure + simple have chosen to have cosmetic surgery. When they do, I stress the importance of a good pre- and postoperative program. Skin care should be as gentle as possible and contain the purest ingredients. Keep in mind that incisions to the capillaries and nerve endings impede circulation. After the capillary network has been cut, full restoration is no longer attainable, often leaving the skin that the network fed dull and sallow.

PEELS

Peels are an excellent way to combat fine lines and dull skin and to keep skin bright and youthful. However, intense, deep peels can have a negative affect on the skin's acid mantle and may require lengthy recovery time.

Your choice of deep peels or gentler, daily peeling treatments depends on your skin type and the results you expect. Sea-salt microdermabrasion "sandblasts" the skin using natural salts and can concentrate on problem areas while performing a gentler abrasion on sensitive skin. It also promotes collagen and elastin production. Whatever peel you use, it must be followed with rich, moisturizing protection. Without this, the newly peeled skin will dehydrate when exposed to the elements.

LASERS

Laser therapy uses light to penetrate 2,940 nanometers or more into the skin. This is deep in comparison to other light treatments on the market. Lasers are very effective in rejuvenating, resurfacing, and correcting skin imperfections. These aggressive treatments work on and below the skin to modify its architecture, heal sun damage, and increase collagen content.

Plasma lasers are intense and very painful. Because light therapy and lasers wound the skin and apply heat, you will experience a powerful burning sensation while undergoing these treatments. Ample recovery time is needed; a twenty-minute treatment requires several days of downtime. The skin is both tender and burnt-looking during the recuperation period. Pixelated or fractionated lasers are less intense, but they do not provide the same dramatic results.

As with the filler market, this sector is advancing so rapidly that it is important to research the latest options if you are considering this route.

PHOTOFACIALS

Photofacials use intense pulsed light (IPL) therapy (with a penetration of 560 to 1,064 nanometers) to promote collagen and elastin production. They are considered a less invasive alternative to lasers, because IPL treatments do not require any downtime, and while treatments may be uncomfortable, they are much less painful. Some clients have described the feeling as similar to having a rubber band snapped against the skin. Personally, I feel it is like a subtle zap of heat and find the accompanying flash of light more of a jolt than the tactile sensation. Because IPL offers variation in light area spot size, beams, time between pulses, and so on, this treatment offers much versatility, and its results can be impressive.

Photofacials are good for treating fine lines and for toning, but they are not as effective for deep wrinkles. I once went to a seminar on light therapy and medical esthetics where the speaker proposed that deep lines be treated with Botox paired with a filler, while the rest of the skin be rejuvenated with IPL. Though this may offer dramatic results, it means loosing a grocery cart of potentially dangerous procedures on your precious face. Long term, this can compromise the skin tissue and health. Photofacials work extremely well to clear the complexion of signs of aging, because IPL can dissolve pigmented lesions and broken capillaries. I have not yet seen any side effects, though blisters, burning, and swelling may occur. Before, during, and after IPL treatments, you must nurture your skin and protect it from the sun. A series of treatments is necessary to achieve the desired results, and the number depends on how advanced the problem being treated is, the condition of your skin, and how zealous you want to be in attaining your goals. While IPL may require more treatments than laser therapy (at a lesser intensity), I always advocate a more cautious, gradual approach.

LIGHT-EMITTING DIODE THERAPY

Light-emitting diode (LED) is another form of light therapy, but it is less intense than IPL. It is almost painless and does not emit the thermal heat that IPL and lasers do, making it much less invasive with little risk of irritation, burning, or swelling. LED energy stimulates tissue repair, promotes skin restoration, and is excellent for healing wounds. Many machines emphasize different colored lights for different functions (such as blue light to kill bacteria and red light to increase collagen production), and time durations differ from machine to machine. An individualized program and a series of treatments are required for optimal results. LED panels like tanning beds are more effective than handheld devices as they provide more energy.

ENDERMOLOGIE

Endermologie is a machine-driven face treatment that uses manual stimulation to regenerate collagen, elastin, and connective tissue. The first step is lymphatic drainage, which is excellent for taking down in-flammation and reducing puffiness and edema (water retention). This is done with a small handheld suction device that is connected to the machine and then placed on the skin and dotted over the skin. The endermologie machine itself automates the pressure and rhythm of the suction. The next step is tissue rejuvenation, in which the pressure is increased. The results you get with this option are subtle and do not match those of a face lift.

COSMETIC ACUPUNCTURE

Acupuncture is wonderful as a cosmetic treatment because it is results-oriented as well as holistic. Using the meridians and points of the body to stimulate circulation and energy flow is a great way to aid total body health and promote a more youthful complexion. Cosmetic acupuncture stimulates collagen and elastin, removes energetic blockages, and treats the internal organs. This treatment is very safe and it requires no pre- or postcare. Cosmetic acupuncture is excellent for treating fine lines and creating more firmness in the complexion. Treatments should be done weekly for a minimum of ten weeks to see a reduction in the appearance of wrinkles.

NONSURGICAL FACE LIFTS

The nonsurgical face lift uses electrodes/electronic currents to stimulate and tone the facial muscles. This treatment, which has received much exposure due to celebrity testimonials, is another great, noninvasive way to treat sagging skin and jowls. Unlike a surgical face lift, however, these treatments can only aid subtle signs of aging, and a series of treatments is required. Even after one treatment, the skin will look brighter as well as feel and appear firmer and tighter. Results last from two weeks to one month. This is a very safe treatment that requires no downtime.

Ayurvedic Solutions for Rejuvenation

Ayurveda views aging as the time when the body has greater tissue loss than gain. This is due to increased vata (depletion of matter) and the accumulation of metabolic waste that inhibits cellular regeneration.

We've already discussed the stages of life, how aging affects the skin, and vata's influence in maturity. As we move through our lives, regardless of our constitution, we all accumulate movement and vata energy, which is why we all begin to show signs of increased vata. Increased vata makes us more conceptual, spiritual, reflective, and willing to explore our connection to the universe, although we still need to mitigate excess vata so we do not become overly depleted and delicate.

Like with vata pacification during menopause, vata-reducing antiaging practices include oiling your body and scalp with sesame oil; eating moist, warm foods; getting ample rest; and engaging in soothing physical and mental activities like yoga and meditation. But nourishment is not the only component to ayurveda's antiaging approach. Cleansing and detoxification are also important. As we age, our systems slow down and so does the process of tissues purging waste on their own. When this occurs, stagnation impedes energetic movement, circulation, and absorption. Habitual detoxification becomes a necessity. For this reason, panchakarma—a special ayurvedic method of intense detoxification—is said to be integral in maintaining youthful vibrancy.

Panchakarma is a multiple-day (in some cases, multiple-week) cleanse that includes a cleansing diet; oiling and steaming the body daily; and five purifying measures. *Panchakarma* means "five actions," referring to *basti* (medicated enemas for evacuating excess vata); *virechana* (gentle laxatives for purging excess pitta); *vama* (vomiting therapy for eliminating excess kapha); *nasya* (administrating medicines through the nasal passages); and bloodletting. Like a body "tune-up," this cleansing process flushes out excess dosha and removes waste from the tissues and gastrointestinal tract. But panchakarma is an intensive and highly-individualized process, so it should be taken on under the guidance of an ayurvedic practitioner or doctor.

Panchakarma detoxification should be coupled with rasayana therapy. Rasayana is a branch of ayurvedic medicine that concentrates on rejuvenation. It ensures the health of the tissues and supports the body's replenishment after panchakarma has removed toxins and emptied the body of waste. It is also used after any surgical procedure to help regenerate the tissues following invasion and incision and to promote overall well-being. Ayurveda does not believe in cleansing or removing damaged tissue without replenishing and nourishing afterward to avoid a relapse. Methods of rasayana include prescribing specific herbs, foods, and practices.

Though rasayana is a supportive, regenerative measure can also be done without doing panchakarma first. Rasayana herbs are packed with antioxidants and help promote cellular growth. They include shatavari, ashwagandha, amalaki, haritaki, guduchi, tulsi, and shilajit. These herbal remedies repair skin, muscle, and bone; restore bodily fluids; and help keep the mind astute and clear. Rasayana therapy also includes incorporating specific foods into your diet; ghee, dates, figs, almonds, green lentils, lemons, and ginger are prescribed for their fortifying properties that replenish and gently cleanse the body. Chyavanprash is a wonderful rasayana food. This nutritive jam is made primarily of amalaki but also includes a plethora of other nourishing ingredients like ghee, honey, haritaki, and pippali. Chyavanprash (also spelled chyawanprash) contains all six tastes of sweet, salty, bitter, astringent, spicy, and sour to balance vata, pitta, and kapha. Preparations from different manufacturers vary, but they are all tridoshic and serve to strengthen the body, protect against stress, and stimulate proper digestion and metabolism.

Like most aspects of ayurveda, healing through rasayana is not limited to what you ingest; it also includes your mental, emotional, and spiritual practices. Your outlook and behavior greatly impact your physical body (and vice versa), and ayurveda outlines seven rasayanas for addressing how to live. The seven rasayana behaviors include speaking the truth; staying free of anger; being respectful of those who impart wisdom (such as teachers, elders, and gurus); gaining Vedic knowledge; practicing meditation; eating rasayana food; and surrounding yourself with like-minded individuals who are also seeking wisdom, groundedness, and enlightenment. These principles shape the ayurvedic viewpoint of how to live and interact with others, and they are said to create blissfulness and longevity.

ANTIAGING PRACTICES FOR EACH DOSHA

Vata is not the only dosha we need to consider when we talk about ayurvedic antiaging practices. As we mature, any of our untreated energetic imbalances worsen and continue to build up. This is why body awareness is so important. Because we have a tendency to accumulate the doshic energies of our predominant dosha, pittas may experience excess heat, acid, and inflammation as they age; kaphas may have water retention and dampness; and vatas may experience intense depletion and tissue loss.

Beautywise, as pittas age, redness and broken capillaries become more apparent. They are prone to inflammation that not only damages collagen and elastin and creates free radicals, but also translates into hypersensitive skin. Topically, it is imperative for pittas to use a mineral sunblock every day to protect the skin from excess inflammation and sun damage. Pittas are the most prone of the three doshas toward hyperpigmentation and freckling that becomes more pronounced as they mature. Because of pittas' skin sensitivity, those who are predominant in this dosha must be careful when using peels. While at-home exfoliation will keep this skin type clear and renewed, concentrated professional peels must be undertaken with caution. Any treatment that may promote redness has the potential to worsen broken and dilated capillaries as well as promote tissue damage. This also pertains to laser and IPL treatments; but these are some of the only methods that remove the appearance of broken blood vessels. They should be done only after a thorough assessment by a highly experienced professional. LED treatments may be a better option for pittas seeking antiaging results; these treatments coupled with an anti-inflammatory skin care regimen comprise a more gentle, gradual form of skin rejuvenation.

Kaphas age the best of all three constitutions, because they naturally have thicker, oilier skin. But kaphas also have a tendency to gain weight as they age and are prone to deep wrinkles made more pronounced by water retention and puffiness. Kaphas benefit most from treatments such as peeling and light therapy. Their skin is innately hardy and can withstand deep peels and sea-salt microdermabrasion. This dosha is also prone to stagnation, so kaphas benefit from the stimulation that LED, IPL, lasers, and nonsurgical face lifts provide. As this skin type ages, it often becomes dull. When a series of peels, sea-salt microdermabrasion, or light therapy is used, circulation is increased, resulting in more radiant-looking skin.

Kaphas usually opt for lighter, less oily skin care products, but they need richer moisturizers as they age to provide better protection. Cream or lotion should be used along with a serum that stimulates circulation in the skin. Products containing vitamin C, ginseng, and sesame oil are ideal.

Vatas have skin that ages easily. People with a vata prakruti may experience overwhelming vata excess, with premature signs of aging.

Symptoms such as loss of muscle and bone mass, thinning skin (so it appears papery and translucent), dehydration, and fine lines are common for this constitution. Vata skin must be protected with heavy creams and oils, using both an oil and a cream—one over the other— as skin matures. Because of vata skin's delicacy, it can only tolerate light peels that promote cell turnover and help thicken skin tissue. Vatas must be careful not to overpeel, dehydrate, or compromise the skin's acid mantle.

This proactive yet conservative approach should be used in conjunction with light therapy. IPL and LED both stimulate collagen production. However, a professional must examine the skin after each treatment and track its progress to ensure that the invasiveness of these techniques does not damage this fragile skin type.

Vatas who also have a strong secondary influence of pitta are highly prone to pigmentation, because the dry quality of this dosha encourages the strengthening of fire and heat energy. Sunblock is essential to vata-pittas, and this is another skin type that requires caution when considering a series of peels, laser therapy, or IPL treatments.

Hyperpigmentation: An Overview

Hyperpigmentation is a common sign of aging. The term generally refers to skin discoloration, and it takes many forms, such as lesions, freckles, and uneven skin tone. This is a growing concern in the beauty industry due to the ever-increasing power of the sun and the increase in inflammation caused by our environment and lifestyle, which causes hyperpigmentation.

Pigmented spots are not limited to mature skin; they can also occur in younger skin, caused by skin damage from inflammation. They most often emerge with age because this damage often takes years to appear.

The Darkness Explained

The skin's color is determined by the amount of melanin it possesses. Melanin (pigment) is produced by melanocytes that are found in the epidermis. The more active your melanocytes, the darker your skin will be.

Structurally, a melanocyte has been compared to an octopus. The melanocyte contains pod-shaped organelles called melanosomes that hold particles of melanin within them. These pods are created and passed through the octopus-like arms of the melanocyte to the keratinocytes (the cells that make up 90 percent of the epidermis). It is here that they gain color. When this process becomes overactive, hyperpigmentation is visible. Ultraviolet rays and other factors cause over- and underactivity of melanocytes, creating lighter and darker patches.

Keratinocytes have a life span of two to three weeks compared to "rogue" melanocytes, which can live for several years. This demonstrates how long a pigmentation issue can persist.

People with sensitive skin are more susceptible to discoloration, because redness and inflammation turn brown over time. While UV rays directly promote dysfunction in melanocytes, the inflammation caused by sunburn also causes discoloration. Scarring is a classic example of inflammation becoming pigmentation. Other triggers are trauma, heat, internal imbalances, poor diet, medication, topical irritants, and improper skin care. Hyperpigmentation is usually a gradual process, only becoming visible years after the damage has occurred.

Genetics are definitely a factor in this condition. Western scientists say people with the "redhead gene" are five times more susceptible to freckling and melanomas. This is due to an abundance of pheomelanin (pink skin pigment); upon UV exposure, pheomelanin produces free radicals. This gene does not necessarily dictate red hair—just a potential for it. Red hair is a characteristic of pitta, which is the ayurvedic dosha responsible for pigmentation.

Eumelanin is a black/brown pigment. During tanning, eumelanin absorbs the energy of light without creating free radicals, thus protecting the skin. It is believed that people with darker skin trace their ancestry to places where more sun exposure has created a need for the skin to protect itself with extra pigment. This pigment is a natural form of SPF. Nevertheless, darker skin easily becomes discolored after burning because of its active melanocytes, while fair skin becomes red and inflamed.

Since the amino acid tyrosine stimulates eumelanin production, many chemical treatments for hyperpigmentation inhibit tyrosine. But once treatments stop, the pigmentation returns.

CAUSES OF HYPERPIGMENTATION

Hyperpigmentation is caused by inflammation from pitta, which governs all action, digestion, metabolism, and assimilation. The transfer of melanin to keratinocytes is governed by this fire dosha, and when pitta is excessive and dysfunctional, this transfer process also becomes irregular. UV damage is simply the skin's inability to digest the sun's heat, while liver spots are due to excess fire stored in this pitta-governed organ. Pigmentation does have genetic influences (primarily based on prakruti), but it is mostly due to the lifestyle choices you make.

The first and easiest way to prevent hyperpigmentation is by using sun protection. Wear a natural mineral sunblock every day without fail. Also be careful not to create photosensitivity in your skin through excessive peeling. Many people with acne become pigmented from the overuse of chemical peeling agents. These individuals likely already had a pitta imbalance that caused their blemishes and skin eruptions, so the addition of deep peels makes them even more vulnerable to discoloration. If they also take antibiotics for their acne, the heating effects of these medications contribute further to hyperpigmentation. Antibiotics increase pitta and dehydrate the skin, which is another cause of discoloration.

Inflammation from hot temperatures also produces hyperpigmentation. Many people know they must use sunblock, but they don't realize they must protect themselves from thermal heat as well. I have had many clients who wear an SPF while outdoors and still get erythema (red skin). This is because they did not avoid heat exposure. Even if you stay in the shade, if the temperatures outside are so high that they make you turn red, this too will contribute to hyperpigmentation.

All inflammation leads to skin discoloration, and because sensitive skin is prone to irritation, this skin type has the highest tendency to pigment. Sensitivity is increased by dehydration, so if you color easily, you need to bolster your skin's water content. The role of hydration is so important that it has been my observation that simply applying better moisturizers reduces pigmentation darkness. Though the change is not dramatic, this indicates that long-term replenishment can treat hyperpigmentation. This has been supported by Dr. Vasant Lad, who states that pigmentation may also be due to a vata corruption in the rakta dhatu (red blood cells). While the blood is governed by pitta, a vata dysfunction within this pitta environment can cause pigmented lesions. Pitta is the most important dosha to address when treating or preventing hyperpigmentation, but it is also necessary to manage vata. Making sure that the skin does not become dehydrated, ensuring that the internal organs are kept moist and lubricated, and paying close attention to your water intake and bowel movements are all necessary. The drier you are, the more fire can flourish within you, and an increase in vata can sometimes "push" an imbalance in pitta.

Digestion is another factor in hyperpigmentation. When your digestive system is weakened and overworked, the inflammation this causes leads to pigmentation. As with acne and rosacea (discussed in the last chapter), eating a pitta-pacifying diet and avoiding any food sensitivities can help support digestion.

Hormones play a large role in hyperpigmentation. Many pregnant women experience changes in skin color, from pigmentation on their abdomen (the stretching of the skin causes inflammation) to what is known as the "pregnancy mask" on their face (caused by hormonal changes). Because melanin production is powered by melanocyte-stimulating hormone (MSH), it is no wonder that the endocrine system influences hyperpigmentation. Remember that pitta governs hormones. Adrenal stress, along with imbalances in estrogen and progesterone, can lead to pigmentation problems.

CONVENTIONAL SOLUTIONS

Peeling with retinol cream or a chemical agent is the most common solution. Naturally derived lactic acid is one of the best ingredients for breaking up pigmentation, provided it is in a natural base. Lactic acid—especially in high concentrations—must be used in conjunction with sun protection, because all peels dehydrate the skin and increase photosensitivity. The skin cannot heal properly when it's dehydrated, so always follow a peel with a nourishing natural moisturizer.

Another conventional solution is bleaching. While effective in inhibiting pigmentation, this can be harsh on sensitive skin and extremely bad for overall health. For example, hydroquinone, a mainstream bleaching agent, has been identified as a carcinogen.

CHEMICAL-FREE SOLUTIONS

Natural solutions are also beneficial, but your expectations must be reasonable. For instance, collagen is fantastic for restoring the skin's moisture levels. It can even fade scars if they are still in their new, red state. But older pigmentation is darker and cannot be eliminated altogether.

Oils like borage and rose hip help skin regeneration and yield excellent results with discoloration. One of my clients said that the darkness of her pigmented spots decreased by approximately a third after using rose hip oil daily for three years. While this may not seem dramatic, keep in mind that this form of treatment involves no peels or bleaching. Natural solutions can improve the appearance of hyperpigmentation but usually do not get rid of it completely.

Engaging in a program of gentle repair coupled with more technological treatments is a better option if you have more ambitious expectations. IPL is extremely effective for diminishing uneven pigmentation (even freckles), but it requires more time and a greater financial investment. Light energy stimulates the body to heal itself and increases collagen production. You need to boost your skin's immunity before treatment, and use a calming, cooling skin care regimen during the treatment series. Afterward, you should focus on adopting a restorative and protective beauty routine.

LED therapy is another excellent treatment for pigmentation. This low-intensity light repairs the skin and stimulates collagen production. It is used for healing during skin cancer therapies and provides safe support for your hyperpigmentation program. While it can be used on its own, results are not as quick as with IPL. LED is most effective when used after peeling or IPL therapy.

From an ayurvedic perspective, hyperpigmentation requires a reduction in excess pitta by internal cooling. Remember, all transformation is governed by pitta. Intense pitta detoxification can be achieved through panchakarma, which begins by loosening pitta toxins through oiling the body externally and internally. The oleation ritual done in preparation of panchakarma is performed through days of oil massage as well as through taking oils internally. This "ripens" the body and brings all excess pitta toxins to their original site—the small intestine—to be cleared out.

Oiling is followed by intense, steam-induced sweating for several days, then pitta toxins are purged with gentle laxatives such as castor oil, aloe vera, Triphala, or prunes. This regimen is very effective in decreasing pigmentation.

If you do not want to take on panchakarma, eating pitta-pacifying foods is also helpful. Incorporate foods into your diet that are sweet or bitter to bring down heat. Leafy greens and celery are excellent bitters. In this instance, *sweet* does not mean sugary; it refers to naturally sweet foods like peas, squash, sweet potatoes, apples, melons, and berries. The word also often means bland and refers to foods that neutralize heat and spice, such as basmati rice, oats, dairy, and avocados. Knowing what to cut out of your diet is also important, and I advise my pigmentation-prone clients to avoid coffee (all caffeine), hot peppers, garlic, radishes, tomatoes, deep-fried dishes, and anything barbequed. Though this may not decrease the appearance of pigmentation, it does help prevent it from becoming worse.

Detoxifying the liver is also key in clearing away excess pitta. As mentioned previously, this can be done by eating a cooling diet and taking liver cleansing herbs such as neem and milk thistle.

Skin tags, or benign skin growths, are by-products of excess pitta (along with kapha accumulation). Often darker in color than normal skin, they disrupt a smooth, even complexion. To diminish the appearance of skin tags, both pitta and kapha need to be decreased.

Even though all these measures are helpful, prevention is always the best practice. This is especially true of hyperpigmentation. Year-round sun protection is essential, as is keeping the skin hydrated. Using products with restorative ingredients—such as collagen, elastin, borage, and rose hip oil—supports the skin and boosts immunity. Strong immunity can prevent disease even when you are in contact with all the causative variables. Avoiding skin trauma, whether in the form of irritation, burns, allergic reactions, or scarring from improper healing, is most important.

Conscious Beauty

Whether you are trying to treat hyperpigmentation, fine lines, or sagging skin, your approach needs to be health-oriented. Antiaging is not about stopping the aging process; it's about using these signs to understand what is happening within. Antiaging is about preventing the deterioration of tissue, and caring for yourself holistically is the only way to keep a vibrant complexion, because your skin's condition is tied to your overall health. The treatments and skin care described in this chapter minimize the signs of aging, but they are only supports to a larger way of living.

This goes beyond eating well and exercising; real antiaging encompasses mind, body, and spirit. The more conscious you are, the more vital and healthy you are. You maintain your youthfulness when you perceive the world around you as new and exciting, and this "youth" stems from a lightness of being and an appreciation of the present. Real antiaging is about not allowing yourself to become dull or stagnant, letting go the past, and being unafraid of the future. This mindset creates self-awareness and enlightenment and encourages you to become more attuned to your body and its imbalances.

With this attitude, you love and accept yourself, making it difficult for your constitution to accumulate blockages or dysfunctions. This is the true definition of beauty.

Conclusion

I hope that, having read this book, you now share my passion for natural skin care as it inspires a new concept of beauty. In this modern age, we must change our old definition to one that fits the world we live in and benefits our society.

To me, beauty is a feeling. While it means different things to different people, I describe it as "good health," which makes us radiate vibrancy and fullness. When we see beauty, we experience awe.

I remember overhearing a conversation about the Northern Lights in my doctor's office. The receptionist was talking to one of the other patients about having seen them, and she said it was the most beautiful experience she'd ever had. Whenever she is depressed, she remembers that vision and feels her spirits lift.

Whether it is found in a person, a place, or an object, beauty is something weighted with a sense of happiness, contentedness, and purpose in living. When we feel beautiful, we feel grounded and confident enough to face the world with happiness and pride. Many people are so desperate for this feeling that they will undertake dangerous procedures to possess it. Such practices are never really effective in the long term, because they are based on an unhealthy idea of beauty and impossible expectations.

Beauty has always been a reflection of cultural norms and values. It is symbolic of who we want to be and what we admire. In the agrarian age, beauty was about youth and fertility. Robustness and stamina were prized because they represented the ability to procreate and contribute to the community's survival. Traces of this view still exist as a biological predisposition. As civilization progressed, society began to appreciate full-bodied women who showed no aptitude for manual work, reflecting leisure-class status. These divergent views show how much beauty is about a desired lifestyle rather than the physical magnetism of an ideal.

With the coming of the industrial age, people accepted a more manufactured idea of beauty. The productivity of standard rules for the legal system, workplace, and consumer goods was reflected in a standardized view of beauty. It became associated with mannequin-like faces and sculpted, cookie-cutter bodies. We are still very much in this era, which is why many women wish for more chiseled features, longer legs, and tinier waists to match society's conventional tastes.

But there are signs that we are entering a more knowledge-focused age in which we must change our definition of beauty just as we are changing our values. With new social issues, new threats to our survival, and new technology, we must align our views of what is attractive and desirable to reflect our new culture.

Beauty must become an embodiment of wisdom, consciousness, and self-empowerment. This supports a move toward a less excessive, less uncompromising, and more inclusive definition. This is why I hope this book becomes a useful part of how we can improve the way we live. It promotes not only clear skin and a healthy body, but also self-respect and a positive perspective of beauty.

Change must come from us first. We often think society must do the

changing, forgetting that collectively we *are* society. It is our responsibility to help change general beliefs and get rid of the self-sabotaging
ones.

This understanding came to me while I was listening to the radio.
There was a discussion about pornography's influence on sexual roles
in our society. The speaker, who had written a book on the subject,
stressed how much the sex industry has shaped what we think of as
"sexy," because so many young people look to Internet pornography
as a guide to sexual dynamics. He described these dynamics as mi-
sogynistic and stated that this would have long-term repercussions on
women's self-image. More interesting, he introduced the finding that
some women believed pornography to be empowering because it as-
serted female desirability. He thought this reflected the dysfunction
of female roles in our society and stated, "Any woman knows beauty is
fleeting in our society, as it is considered synonymous with youth. If a
woman cannot sustain sexual attractiveness through maturity, the idea
of power through sex is a fallacy."

This spurred an epiphany for me: it is often women who accept
these images and promote them to each other. Yet when dominated
by this youthful, pornographic image, we can never feel beautiful
from middle age on. It is up to us to change this social norm to a more
positive one. Because I do not believe beauty is about being perfectly
proportioned, I have found women attractive because of the power in
their voices; I have found men attractive because of the beauty of their
intentions; and I have found myself to be most beautiful when I am living my life in a holistic way.

So I hope this book gives you not only the tools and knowledge
you need to maintain your body, but also an understanding of how
subtle, healthy practices can yield powerful and positive outcomes.
Beauty, as an intangible feeling of being comfortable in your own skin,

affects how you conduct yourself. If you feel ugly or out of balance, you may not be in the right headspace to be open-minded, unselfish, and positive.

A change in the definition of beauty is a change in the way we view our world. We must commit ourselves to this responsibility. I see people gravitating toward it already. It is not my movement; it is a natural change that resonates with many individuals. Pure + simple has been successful not only because natural skin care is in vogue, but because it is a company that aligns itself with the way its customers want to live.

I believe the Pure + simple concept involves both a method of self-care and a lifestyle. This new cultural phenomenon is about respect for others, the environment, and ourselves. It is about a world where ideas will be more valuable than goods and where status will come through societal contribution instead of an accumulation of wealth. It is a change that must happen if we are going to ensure the health of our communities.

The future is ambiguous, but I have faith that we will enter an age of consciousness and flexibility, when the old, rigid norms become outdated and inapplicable. Beauty, as superficial as people may consider it, is central to this change, because beauty is really about embodying what we value.

Beauty made pure and simple makes me excited for the future.

Glossary

ama: Toxins found within the body. In ayurveda, ama is a result of improper digestion or assimilation, leading to unprocessed waste.

antioxidant: An ingredient in beauty care products that inhibits oxidation of and free radical damage to skin cells. Antioxidants are primarily used in antiaging products.

Ashwagandha: A root herb used in ayurvedic medicine to pacify vata and kapha. Ashwagandha is also referred to as Indian ginseng or winter cherry, and it helps with many nervous system ailments as well as tissue degeneration.

candida: A fungus found primarily in the gut, digestive tract, mouth, and genitals. While candida exists normally within the body, an excess can contribute or lead to a variety of illnesses and conditions (for example, acne).

carcinogen: A substance or an action that has been found to cause cancer.

dermatitis: Any skin inflammation, including allergic reactions and rashes.

dermis: One of the three layers of the skin. Located beneath the epidermis, it is responsible for hydrating the skin and contains collagen and elastin molecules.

doshas: The three energetic influences of ayurveda that make up individual constitutions. The doshas are vata (air), pitta (fire), and kapha (water/earth); they can also be used to describe the qualities of substances and foods.

eczema: A common skin disorder that takes a variety of forms (inflammation, itchiness, flakiness, redness, and bacterial lesions).

endocrine disrupter: Any substance or action that leads to an imbalance in the hormonal system.

epidermis: The surface layer of the skin. It is composed mainly of keratinocytes.

estrogen: A hormone found in both men and women, but primarily linked with the female reproductive system. Estrogen plays a role in the texture as well as the hydration of the skin due to its support of hyaluronic acid.

eumelanin: The type of melanin (pigment) found in skin and hair that imparts a brown or black color.

extraction: The physical removal of dried oil that causes clogged pores and blemishes. Extractions are best performed by a professional esthetician as part of a facial.

ghee: Clarified butter used in ayurveda as a vehicle for medicines and alone as a healing agent. Ghee is used primarily in food preparation, but it can also be applied topically for its anti-inflammatory properties.

glycolic acid: An ingredient found in cosmetic preparations that peel and exfoliate the skin.

gommage: An exfoliating treatingment that is applied like a mask and is rubbed off when dry. This rubbing or rolling off action is what enables exfoliation.

guduchi: A climbing vine used as a medicinal herb to rejuvenate the pitta and vata doshas. It is considered a rasayana that nourishes the body's tissues and creates mental clarity.

hypodermis: The deepest layer of the skin, found under the dermis. This fatty tissue serves as a cushion to the body and its internal organs.

intense pulsed light (IPL) therapy: A beauty treatment that uses high-intensity pulses of light to promote collagen production and diminish the look of broken capillaries and hyperpigmentation; it is also popularly used for permanent hair removal and reduction. IPL usually requires no downtime for recovery and is much less painful than laser therapy.

kapha: One of the three doshas described in ayurveda kapha is characterized by the elements of earth and water. It governs the qualities of heaviness, slowness, stability, and wetness. It is also responsible for retention, accumulation, and growth.

keratinocytes: Cells that comprise 90 percent of the epidermis (top layer of skin).

laser treatment: The use of deeply penetrating light rays to stimulate collagen production, broken capillaries, and pigmented lesions. Lasers are more intense than IPL; they aim to accomplish many of the same beauty goals, are more invasive, and also garner faster and more dramatic results. Unlike IPL, laser treatment requires several days for recovery and includes topical side effects such as temporary burn marks and skin discomfort.

light-emitting diode (LED) therapy: The use of low-intensity light to kill bacteria and to repair and heal tissue.

lymphatic system: The network consisting of lymphoid tissue, lymph fluid, and the vessels that move and transport that fluid within the body. Water retention is often attributed to a buildup of lymph fluid. Lymphoid tissue is related to the body's immune function, as it contains white blood cells (lymphocytes) that protect against and combat disease.

melanin: The pigment in the skin that determines its color.

melanocytes: Cells that produce melanin and dictate the skin's pigment.

melanosome: An organelle that holds particles, or "packets," of melanin.

These particles are created and passed on to keratinocytes (in the epidermis) by melanocytes.

mineral makeup: A type of makeup that uses all-natural minerals (such as zinc oxide and titanium dioxide) in its formulation.

organic: Cultivated without the use of chemical pesticides.

petrolatum: A petrochemical used as a base in many beauty preparations. Petroleum has been identified as a cause of clogged pores and acne breakouts, as well as liver and kidney abnormalities via its absorption through the skin.

pheomelanin: The type of melanin (pigment) found in skin and hair that imparts a red or pink color.

pitta: One of the three doshas described in ayurveda, pitta is characterized by the element of fire. It governs the qualities of inflammation, heat, and sharpness. It is also responsible for transformation and digestion.

pranayama: The act of controlling breath for balancing and healing purposes. These breathing exercises and techniques are often part of yogic and ayurvedic regimens to calm the mind, detoxify the respiratory system, and increase oxygen intake and *prana* (life force).

progesterone: A cooling hormone that plays an important role in the functions of the female body and reproductive system.

psoriasis: A skin condition characterized by inflammation and flakiness. It is also considered to be one of the more serious beauty ailments because it is an autoimmune disease.

rasayana: A substance or an action that rejuvenates the mind, body, and spirit. Rasayanas can serve as antiaging tools, as they support the immune system and repair the body's tissues.

rosacea: A skin condition characterized by redness, broken capillaries, and sometimes pustules. Western medicine and ayurveda consider rosacea to be a cardiovascular disorder that is aggravated by anything that stimulates the circulatory system.

sea-salt microdermabrasion: An exfoliating beauty treatment that involves "sandblasting" the skin with all-natural sea-salt crystals. This type of microdermabrasion is employed to treat acne, acne scarring, and signs of aging.

Shatavari: An ayurvedic herb used to calm excess vata and pitta and to promote kapha. Shatavari is known for its support of the reproductive system and its ability to increase fertility. It is also used as a nourishing agent that aids in muscle and weight gain.

sodium laurel sulfate (SLS): A chemical detergent used in beauty care products such as soaps, body washes, shampoos, and toothpastes. It is very harsh and strips the skin's natural oils. It is also linked to tissue malformation, impaired healing, and increased absorption of other toxic chemicals.

SPF (sun protection factor): A measurement that indicates how long a given product or ingredient allows skin to be exposed to ultraviolet rays before burning. For example, a product with SPF 10 allows a person to stay in the sun ten times longer without burning than he or she could without the product.

testosterone: A heat/inflammation-causing hormone that often contributes to acne.

tridoshic: An ayurvedic term used to describe a substance that treats all three doshas or an individual who possesses all of them in equal proportions.

Triphala: An ayurvedic preparation that combines three fruits (amalaki, bibhitaki, and haritaki) to aid detoxification and balance all three doshas. It is one of the most important ayurvedic medicines and is most often taken in powder form.

turmeric: An anti-inflammatory, antibacterial root herb, also known as curcumin. Turmeric is used in ayurvedic medicine for treating all three doshas and is most often found as a powder or in capsules.

Sometimes whole or fresh turmeric can be found, but this is rare in North America.

vata: One of the three doshas described in ayurveda, vata is characterized by the element of air. It governs the qualities of dryness, lightness, and roughness. It is also responsible for movement.

Rejuvenating Resources

Natural Skin Care Brands

Dr. Hauschka Skin Care
20 Industrial Dr. East
South Deerfield, MA 01373
http://drhauschka.com
This company offers a full range of
natural/organic face care, body care,
and hair care, as well as some internal
supplements.

Jurlique Skin Care
2425 Colorado Ave., Suite B250
Santa Monica, CA 90404
Phone: 800-854-1110
http://www.jurlique.com
This company offers a full range of
natural/organic face care, body care, hair
care, and essential oils.

Naturopathica
74 Montauk Hwy., Suite 1
East Hampton, NY 11937
Phone: 631-329-2525
http://www.naturopathica.com
This company offers a full range of natu-
ral/organic face care, body care, and hair
care.

Pure + simple
25-2700 Dufferin St.
Toronto, Ontario
M6B 4J3 Canada
Phone: 416-322-9093
http://www.pureandsimple.ca
This company offers a full range of
natural/organic and ayurveda-inspired
face care, body care, and hair care.

Saffron Rouge Organic Beauty
Phone: 866-322-3227
http://www.saffronrouge.com
This company offers a full range of
natural/organic face care, body care,
and hair care.

Ayurvedic Herbs and Supplements

The Ayurvedic Institute
1131 Menaul Blvd. NE
Albuquerque, NM 87112
Phone: 505-291-9698
http://www.ayurveda.com
The online store of this ayurvedic

educational center sells loose ayurvedic and Western medicinal herbs. It retails its own Sidha Soma brand of tinctures, medicated ghees and oils, as well as a number of ayurvedic products from other manufacturers.

Banyan Botanicals
6705 Eagle Rock Ave. NE
Albuquerque, NM 87113
Phone: 800-953-6424
http://www.banyanbotanicals.com
This producer of USDA-certified, organic herbs and remedies sells loose ayurvedic herbs, capsules, massage oils, and other ayurvedic products.

Circle of Health, Inc.
Phone: 541-944-7243
http://www.ayurveda-herbs.com/index.htm
This site has an extensive line of Rasayana jams for treating various ailments.

Himalaya Herbal Healthcare
http://www.himalayahealthcare.com
This site offers a pharmaceutical-grade line of ayurvedic medicines and herbs.

Maharishi Ayurveda Products International (MAPI)
1680 Hwy 1 North, Suite 2200
Fairfield, Iowa 52556
Phone: 800-255-8332
http://www.mapi.com/maharishi_ayurveda.html
This company sells all types of wild-crafted ayurvedic herbal products, from spices and supplement capsules to teas and ghees.

Nature's Formulary
1 Barney Road, Suite 128
Clifton Park, NY 12065
Phone: 800-923-9338
http://www.naturesformulary.com
These organic, wild-crafted ayurvedic supplements and personal care products are available in health food stores as well as online.

Organic India
5311 Western Ave., Suite T
Boulder, CO 80301
Phone: 720-406-3940
http://organicindia.com
This company offers teas, syrups, herbals, capsules, and other ayurvedic foodstuffs.

Ayurvedic Clinics and Wellness Centers

AyurvedaGram Heritage Wellness Centre
Panchakarma Clinic
Bangalore, India
Phone: +91 (80) 656-51090
http://www.ayurvedagram.com

The Ayurvedic Institute
11311 Menaul Blvd. NE
Albuquerque, NM 87112
Phone: 505-291-9698
http://www.ayurveda.com

California Center for Integrative Medicine
9099 Soquel Drive, Cottage 7
Aptos, CA 95003
Phone: 831-662-2997
http://AyurvedicHealing.net

The Chopra Center
2013 Costa del Mar Rd.
Carlsbad, CA 92009
Phone: 760-494-1639
http://www.chopra.com

Kerala Ayurveda
http://ayurvedaonline.com/ayurveda-clinics
This website provides a listing of clinics
that practice Kerala ayurveda.

Natural/Holistic Spas

Naturopathica Holistic Health Spa
74 Montauk Highway, Suite 1
East Hampton, NY 11937
Phone: 631-329-2525
http://www.naturopathica.com/naturo
pathica_spa

Pratima Spa
110 Greene St., Suite 701
New York, NY 10012
Phone: 212-581-8136
http://pratimaspa.com

Pure + simple Spa
2375 Yonge St.
Toronto, Ontario
M4P 2C8 Canada
http://www.pureandsimple.ca

Pure + simple Spa
41 Avenue Rd.
Toronto, Ontario
M5R 2G3, Canada
http://www.pureandsimple.ca

Pure + simple Spa
725 King St. West

Toronto, Ontario
M5V 2W9, Canada
http://www.pureandsimple.ca

Pure + simple Spa
348 Lakeshore Rd. East
Oakville, ON
L6J 1J6, Canada
http://www.pureandsimple.ca

Ra Spa
119 North San Fernando Blvd.
Burbank, CA 91502
http://raorganicspa.com

Ruby Room
1743–45 W. Division St.
Chicago, IL 60622
http://rubyroom.com

Blogs

Holistic Vanity
http://holisticvanity.com
Kristen's own beauty blog is devoted to
ayurveda, wellness, and looking fabulous.

Kerala Ayurveda blog
http://ayurvedaprograms.blogspot.com
This is a resource for all things
ayurveda, including articles about and
recipes for natural healing and wellness.

Ayurvedic Educational Institutions

The Ayurvedic Institute
11311 Menaul Blvd. NE
Albuquerque, NM 87112

Phone: 505-291-9698
http://ayurveda.com
Founded by renowned physician and author Vasant Lad, The Ayurvedic Institute offers full certification programs, short-term seminars, and intensive education sessions.

Kerala Ayurvedic Academy
http://www.ayurvedaacademy.com
With schools all over the United States, Kerala Ayurvedic Academy has some of the most respected ayurvedic physicians as faculty members.

Recommended Reading

Ayurveda: A Practical Guide: The Science of Self-Healing by Vasant Lad (Wilmot, Wis.: Lotus Press, 1985).
This practical guide helps readers self-diagnose their health problems and offers an overview of ayurvedic philosophy and methodology.

Ayurveda for Women by Robert E. Svboda (Rochester, VT: Healing Arts Press, 2000).
This wonderful book focuses on women's bodies and health issues and the role of ayurveda in maintaining a healthy, natural lifestyle.

The Complete Book of Ayurvedic Home Remedies by Vasant Lad (New York: Three Rivers Press, 1999).
This staple resource is a useful addition to any home library.

Perfect Health by Deepak Chopra (New York: Harmony, 2001).
This is a well-written, easy-to-read introduction to ayurvedic science.

Index

constipation
  acne and, 151–52
  dehydration and, 121
contingencies
  ayurveda and, 37–38
  diet, 39–41
  emotional, 42–43
  menstrual cycle, 42
  stage-of-life, 43–45
  time, 40, 42
  weather, 38–39
coriander cold infusion, 176
cortisone, 22
creams, day and night, 87–88
cystic acne ("blind pimples"),
  151–52, 157, 163–64

decongesting, 132–33
  gentle ayurvedic protocol
    for daily, 137–40
  the skin, 133–37
dehydrated skin, 68, 69, 72–75,
  193
  dry, 68, 74
  oily, 68, 70, 72–73, 76–77
dehydration, stress and, 121
deposition (fifth stage of disease), 48
dermis, 67
diazolidinyl urea, 23
diet
  aging, heat, and, 190
  anti-inflammatory, 148–50,
    190
  estrogen, menopause, and,
    192–93
  not eating late at night, 129
  rosacea and, 176
  skin sensitivities and,
    169–70
  See also food
diet contingencies, 39–41
diethanolamine (DEA), 22–23
differentiation/destruction
  (sixth stage of disease), 49
disease, six stages of, 46–49

dispersion (third stage of disease), 48
doshas, 27–29, 37
  antiaging practices for each
    of the, 204–6
  See also kapha; pitta; vata
dry dehydrated skin, 68, 74
dry hydrated skin, 68, 74
drying agents, 108

earth. See kapha
eczema, 167, 181–82, 186
  ayurvedic solutions, 183–86
  triggers for, 182–83
  types of, 183–86
  See also sensitivity
elastin, 194
endermologie, 200–201
Eng, Jean (Kristen Ma's
  mother), 2, 4–5
environmentally-friendly products, 15–17
epidermis, 66
estrogen, 191–94
exercising, 125–26
  early in the day, 130
exfoliation, 95–96, 98, 134–35
extractions, 99, 133–34
eyebrows, 104
eyes
  caring for, 89–93
  dark circles around, 91–92
  puffy, 92
  sensitive, 90–91

face lifts, nonsurgical, 201
face mapping, 49–52
facials, 97–100
fat deposits/cholesterol, 92–93
fillers, injected, 197
fire. See pitta
Firming Eye Gel, 184
food chart, ayurvedic, 39, 41
foods
  hydrating, 110–11
  See also diet

free radical damage, 194–95
frown lines, 53

Galland, Leo, 122
gargling with oil, 139
gender differences in skin, 70–71
groundedness, 130
guduchi, 59

haritaki, 59–60
Hawken, Paul, 16
heart, 57
heat and acne, 147–50
hibiscus tea, 176
hormones and acne, 150–51
hyaluronic acid, 71, 80, 112,
  192, 194
hydrated skin, 73–75
hydrating ingredients, best,
  112–14
hydration
  how to hydrate from the
    outside, 109–10
  increasing, from the inside
    out, 110–11
  maintaining, 107–9
  See also moisturizing
hydrosols, 72, 119
hyperpigmentation, 206
  causes, 208–10
  chemical-free solutions,
    210–13
  conventional solutions, 210
  the darkness explained,
    207–8
hypodermis, 67

imidazolidinyl urea, 23
inflammation, 167
  and acne, 147–50, 157
  and aging, 189–90
  diet and, 148–50, 190
  and hyperpigmentation,
    209–10
  stress and, 123
  See also eczema; rosacea